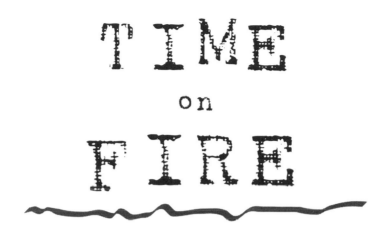

TIME
on
FIRE

My Comedy
of Terrors

by
Evan Handler

An Owl Book
Henry Holt and Company   New York

Henry Holt and Company, Inc.
Publishers since 1866
115 West 18th Street
New York, New York 10011

Henry Holt ® is a registered trademark of
Henry Holt and Company, Inc.

LIBRARY OF CONGRESS CATALOGING-IN-PUBLICATION DATA
Handler, Evan.
Time on fire: my comedy of terrors / by Evan Handler.
p.   cm.
"An Owl book."
1. Handler, Evan—Health.   2. Myelocytic leukemia—Patients—
United States—Biography.   I. Title.
[RC643.H286   1997]   97–1750
362.1´9699419´0092—dc21   CIP
[B]

ISBN 0-8050-5067-1

Henry Holt books are available for special promotions
and premiums. For details contact: Director, Special Markets.

First published in hardcover in 1996
by Little, Brown and Company.

First Owl Book Edition—1997

Everything you read in this book is true.
Some of the names have been changed.

Printed in the United States of America
All first editions are printed on acid-free paper. ∞

3   5   7   9   10   8   6   4   2

CONTENTS

And I will never, ever, ever, ever grow so old again.

— Van Morrison,
"Sweet Thing"

For Murry and Enid;
Lillian and Lowell

. . . old sorrow, written in tears and blood.
A sadly inappropriate gift, it would seem . . .

— Eugene O'Neill, 1941

ACKNOWLEDGMENTS

In addition to the many heroes described or alluded to in the story, there are a number of people who deserve credit for helping this book to become a reality. First and foremost, my gratitude goes to Liz Tuccillo. She encouraged me to start writing, and her support and love and generosity never wavered. She is the hero behind the telling of the story, and for her wisdom and her friendship I will be forever in her debt.

Also instrumental in creating this book were Jackie Reingold and my family: Murry, Enid, Lillian, and Lowell. It was never their choice to expose themselves as I have done, nor would they all agree with everything I've written. Nevertheless, they gave me unlimited access to their recollections and wide license to recount events as I perceived them. Their bravery, both during my illness and today, is astonishing.

Of course I'd like to thank my editors, Catherine Crawford—for her immediate and continued faith in the project—and Darcy Tromanhauser, as well as all the caring professionals at Little, Brown and Company and Henry Holt/Owl Books. I have felt very well taken care of.

The director of my play, who was my very first editor, was Marcia Jean Kurtz. She handled the production, and me, with love, with grace, and with an abundance of talent.

Finally, there are a large number of individuals and organizations who lent their support in all manner of ways. In no particular order, and with apologies to whomever I may have left out, they are:

Naked Angels; Paul Newman and Newman's Own, Inc.; The Corporation of Yaddo; Lisa Kogan; Erica Silverman; Bernard Gersten; Gus Rogerson; Lenore Zerman; Don DeLillo; Larry Kramer; Jeremy Kagan, Michelle Satter, and Sundance Institute; Carole Rothman, Suzanne Davidson, and the Second Stage Theatre; Robert Brustein and the American Repertory Theatre; Kate Ruddon; Shelly Gidamer; Dr. Martin Abeloff; Craig Carlisle; David Eigenberg; Kenneth Lonergan; Beth Emelson; Jenny Peek; Fisher Stevens; Pippin Parker; Rob Morrow; Paul McCrane; Barry Singer; Kay Liberman; Loudon Wain Wright III; David Black; and Susan Raihofer.

TIME on FIRE

CONSCRIPTION

"I'm afraid it is not good news," is what he said. "It is bad news. It is in the bone marrow. It's an acute myelogenous leukemia."

Now, for some reason this doctor, in my memory, has turned into Richard Nixon. If Richard Nixon had ever been interested in acting, in the movie, I'd have given him the part.

We were in this doctor's office for some time after that. My parents, my girlfriend, Jackie, and me. There was some talk of intensive chemotherapy, remission rates; the phrase "not curable" hit me from somewhere. I only remember that I kept rubbing the side of my face, really hard.

"Okay, okay, okay," I finally said, and everyone seemed a little bit startled, as if they'd forgotten I was actually there in the room with them. "I have to get out of here now. We can talk about all this later," and I got up to go.

"I wouldn't wait very long," Dr. Nixon said. And we stumbled out of his office and into the street.

Have you ever had the feeling, after you've been in a movie theater, of being surprised that you're still in the same city that you were before you went inside? Or that it's still daytime; or that you're still the same person, with the same name, in the same life, on the same planet? It was like that, on the corner of Second Avenue and Seventeenth Street in New York. It was ninety-six degrees, and we couldn't get a cab, and we couldn't look at each other either. I heard them muttering, and there was probably even some conversation. Like "Should we walk?" "No. I can't walk." Something like that. But I was afraid that if I looked at them after what had just happened, they would all be complete strangers. Literally. That I wouldn't recognize anyone. Like one of those *Twilight Zone* episodes, where everyone acts like they know you, and they do know all about you, but you've never met a single one of them, and you can't understand how your life got switched around with someone else's, or how to find your way back to your own.

Back at my apartment it was like mission control for the rest of the day. Phone calls going out and coming in. Contacting friends, relatives, and trying to come up with a plan of action. Of course the goal was to find the very best of the best, and through any means possible, to find a world-class treatment center for me. It had to be mid-afternoon by now, and since no one had eaten anything all day, Jackie and my father went out to get Chinese food. My mother was in the kitchen talking to my uncle the oral surgeon on the phone.

I sat on my bed and I cried. Not really cried, I sobbed and I screamed. I broke down in a way that I had never seen an adult go before. I sat in a room, alone, moaning and slobbering for close to an hour. And I had no frame of reference at all. For anything that was happening to me. I was twenty-four years old, and my girlfriend, Jackie, whom I'd been seeing for a year so far, had just moved into my apartment to live with me. I had already been a professional actor for most of the last seven years, and my career seemed like it was really about to take off. I hadn't yet learned how often a career can *seem* to be about to take off. Now I know that there are careers in full flight and those that are constantly threatening to take off. I was very glad that I didn't have one that was firmly earthbound, and I enjoyed my skips and hops up and down the runway, all the while dreaming of orbit. While understudying in the Broadway production, I had just been offered the plummest role in the national tour of Neil Simon's play *Biloxi Blues;* I had a deal worked out to go to Israel for ten weeks to make a film with a renowned West German filmmaker; and I had a meeting scheduled for the following Monday with Warren Beatty for final casting approval on a movie that he was about to make with Dustin Hoffman. Okay, so it turned out to be *Ishtar.* It still would have been better than what I was facing.

The horror of sensing that my life was over wasn't something that my mind could grasp. I'm not even sure that a "life," as a separate entity, really exists. My perception was one of having been robbed, stripped bare, of every possession, liberty, freedom, hope, and dream for the future. If you added those things up, they somehow equaled my life. Maybe I'm a guy who lives with his mind racing ahead into tomorrow more than I should, but I couldn't stop thinking that night about all the dreams and plans I had that might never be. A home, a wife, kids. Having a history to look back on. Becoming the person I wanted to become someday. Anything that I had ever said or thought before that word — "someday." Gone. Not for me. That was my biggest fear at that moment. The absence of a future for which to endure the present.

I felt as if I had wasted enormous amounts of time in my life, and that I had to have a second chance immediately. But first I had to go into the hospital for a month, maybe more. I couldn't even start my new beginning right away. I was going to be exiled from my history, from my future, from time itself, all in the hope of possibly regaining contact with them. Time became a concrete entity to me like never before. Never mind being more aware of it, I could've sculpted with it. I could have cooked it and eaten it. I felt far, far away from everything that made me *me*, I was getting home-sick already, and if there was a journey that had to be made first, I wanted to start now and travel fast.

I didn't calm down one bit until the Hunan Chicken scent hit my nose and the meat started sliding down my throat. There it was, my first lesson in survival: grief gives way to hunger.

I had the urge to tell some people what was happening to me. For instance, my sister and brother. My sister, Lillian, lived in Lancaster, Pennsylvania, with her fiancé and had settled into a rather staid, solid existence as far from my life in New York as one could get. Lowell, my brother, was living a couple of hours north of the city and had been struggling to get work as a photographer. It wasn't that Lowell lacked talent. The trouble was largely due to a neurologi-cal disorder that causes him to twitch and bark in a way that can sometimes frighten people. He's got Tourette syndrome. He likes to call himself a Touretter. The only times he's not twitching are when he's sleeping or having sex. The two activities my brother swears his doctor recommends he engage in as often as possible.

My parents were very understanding of my need to speak to someone, to voice out loud what was happening to me, as a kind of reality check. If I said it to someone and they reacted, then maybe I could begin to fathom that it was really there and get prepared to live it. That kind of thing. But couldn't I just wait to tell my brother until Monday? He had a job, a photo shoot, on Sunday, and, "He needs the work so badly, and it would be a shame to upset him so that he might not do a good job. Yes, why don't you just call Lowell and tell him we don't know anything yet? Then on Monday, after he's through with his job, call him back and tell him you have leukemia."

Wait until Monday. It was now Friday.

At first I agreed, but then I thought, No, wait a minute, god-dammit. I'm calling Lowell and I'm going to tell him and let him make up his own mind what to do.

"Hey, Low'll."

"Evan. Hey, how you doin'?"

"Uh. Not so good, I'm afraid."

"What's the matter?"

"I have leukemia."

"You what?"

"I have leukemia."

"What do you mean you have leukemia?"

"I mean we went to the doctor this morning, and he said I've got leukemia."

"Leukemia?"

"Yeah."

"Holy shit . . ."

My brother is the emotional one in the family. I think that's why my mother was afraid to let him know right away. As if, by waiting until our shock had worn off to tell him, we could avoid having to confront his shock altogether. But, as we expected, he was quite upset, and my parents' worry was immediately doubled. Concern for my brother and his pain was like a reflex to them.

Up until the moment that I called my brother I had always believed mine was the quintessence of the "perfect American family." Like the storybook legend of the Kennedys. Never mind that the Kennedy family history was riddled with tragedy and horror. What mattered was the success. The aura, the admirable credentials. My father had left a childhood of economic and cultural poverty behind in Bangor, Maine, to create a successful career in New York as an illustrator and advertising executive. My mother had prided herself on receiving a master's degree and going to work long before the women's movement popularized the trend. The children in the family had grown up either intellectual or artistic, or both. Like in the Kennedy family, my father had long before instituted guidelines that turned family interactions into pseudo-business transactions. We were paid for performing our household chores but not until we had submitted an itemized bill for the services rendered. If we wanted a raise in our allowance or in our hourly wage, a letter had to be drafted, stating the request and giving reasons to support its necessity. Not that these rules were enforced harshly or without humor. We were all, even as we obeyed them, aware of their absurdity. And for the neighbors it must have been tremendously amusing. It was not an uncommon sight to pass our house and see the three children parading around the front door shouting slogans, with placards in our grimy hands that read "Murry Handler Unfair to Workers — ON STRIKE."

In my apartment, after Dr. Nixon's diagnosis, I was having my first hint of suspicion that my family was anything other than perfect and enviable. Of course there was the solid marriage, and there were the artistic children surrounded by love and encouragement — no small achievements. But I now saw clearly for the first time what lurked beneath. My brother had a serious neurological impairment obvious to all outside our clan; my sister had been isolated from the family for quite a while and was planning to marry a Catholic man, a situation that caused tensions no one would have previously admitted were possible; and I had just been diagnosed with an almost always rapidly fatal disease. I became very conscious that my perception of my family, and our place in the world when we compared ourselves with others (which was what we always did, compare ourselves with others), had never really been as golden as I'd believed, and was certainly, now, anything but blessed.

It didn't take long for us to set our sights on Memorial Sloan-Kettering Cancer Center in New York, and my mother was back on the phone, trying to arrange for my admission that night or the next morning. We had decided on Sloan-Kettering largely because I wanted to stay near my home. I had accumulated a fairly large group of friends over the years and I already expected to need them close by. Once the choice to remain in New York had been made, we were understandably seduced by the mammoth reputation of this renowned institution. We had scouted around and been quoted the name of one particular doctor there by several different sources, and we were proud of ourselves for being such educated consumers. No getting pushed around for us. We checked and double-checked. Asked other doctors about the doctor we were considering. All the signs said step one was going well.

Not that we hadn't been warned at all. We'd been told that life inside Sloan-Kettering could be hard. It's not the place to go to get pampered, I was told by my uncle the oral surgeon, who was doing a lot of the investigating for us. "Sloan-Kettering is a research hospital, and they have a reputation for being a little short on warmth. It's not a summer camp," he said.

I told him, "I'm not looking for a summer camp. I've got leukemia and I want a doctor who's a killer. I want someone who's ruthless. I don't plan on being in there but a short time, anyway."

At eight A.M. the next morning I became patient #865770. Some strings had been pulled to get me admitted to Sloan-Kettering right away, but we were totally unprepared for the bureaucratic Hell that would greet us when we checked in. I guess I had a vision of traffic being stopped on Sixty-eighth Street so the kid with cancer could pass. At least I expected to be treated as someone who was in great emotional pain and about to undergo great physical pain as well. And that's exactly how I was to be treated — New York style.

We were herded — Jackie, my parents, and I — through a maze of corridors that were *packed* with hordes of other people. We passed people in wheelchairs; people with bandages covering their necks, their heads, their faces. Strangely gray-toned people with no hair; people wearing surgical face masks; people, people everywhere. People moaning in pain. Most of the people looked tired and resigned. They seemed to understand that what was happening to them was horrible to no one but themselves.

9

We landed in a deserted waiting room, where we sat for an hour and a half before my name was called. I was then directed to a cubicle, where I faced a very young Puerto Rican woman. There was a lipstick-stained cigarette burning in an ashtray on her desk. The woman immediately began firing ridiculously mundane questions at me in a heavily accented mumble without ever once making eye contact. I thought to myself, Oh, of course. Of course. These people train at the same school as the token booth clerks. I had to ask her to repeat several of the questions over again, and she would become exasperated and heave a huge sigh each time. She hated me. She really hated her job, I guess, but she was acting like she hated me. I wanted her to like me. I was, in fact, heavily invested, emotionally, in having that poor, overworked, disgusted secretary like me. Finally she said something to me that sounded like "Make a buck up to X ray, push a dove in a smocker, and wait for a technician." She pulled a form from her typewriter, handed it to me, and reloaded, all without looking up.

After typing several more lines, she stopped and looked over at me for the first time. Once I had her attention I was so pleased that a big smile broke out across my face. She was quite pretty when she wasn't scowling. Now she was just staring at me blankly. I said, "Thank you."

She sat looking at me like a cow looks at you when you say "moo."

I rode the elevator to another floor where I got better instructions. I was to undress, *put my clothes in a locker,* and wait in another holding pen to have a chest X ray taken. This waiting room was so crowded that I couldn't find a seat, and included rows of people lying on stretchers who stared into that middle distance that only the truly abandoned seem able to see. Another hour or so and I was hustled through the procedure and on my way to the twelfth floor.

The elevator door opened and the noise hit me. A hospital floor is not a quiet place. Bells were ringing, metal carts were clanging, and there were voices constantly blaring over the PA system. Nurses were calling for doctors; patients calling for nurses; nurses calling out instructions to each other. My parents, who had come up while I was waiting for my X ray, came over to meet me.

"You're in twelve twenty-nine," my father said. "Twelve twenty-nine B." And we started down the hallway to find the room. Zigzagging toward us from the far end of the hall was a man wearing blue flannel pajamas, with a bright red fresh incision running from just over one eyebrow all the way to the back of his hairless head. The skin of his scalp was stretched so tightly that a seam was formed along the incision line and his skull was held closed with what looked to be very large staples.

He smiled, and called, "Good morning!" as he passed.

I stole glimpses into some of the rooms as we walked. Most held pairs of beds with older people lying on their backs, very still. Some had either nurses or family members leaning over them, talking quietly or tending to some need.

In the hall were a few younger men and women, pacing in hospital gowns and bathrobes, or huddled with a loved one who wore street clothes, whispering quietly to each other, in poses that reminded me of prisoners plotting escape in B movies.

"Ohhh. Help me. Please. Please help me." A woman alone in a room was crying out. The sound got louder as we passed and faded as we turned the corner. "Please help me . . . please help me." I realized that her voice had been in the background since I got off the elevator. And it was the background music that played all night and day for the next four weeks. "Oh, God . . . please help me."

As we passed the patients' lounge I tried to peer in through the dense haze of smoke and saw a small room, crowded with pasty-looking figures, all hooked up by tubes to bottles dangling from dilapidated, leaning poles on wheels. They were furiously puffing on cigarettes with grim expressions on their faces as they sat on couches with torn orange upholstery. *The Price Is Right* was blasting away at high volume from a TV set that no one was watching.

A madhouse, I thought. I've come to die in a madhouse. We got to Room 1229, and I hurried in as if I was diving for cover. I went right to the bed and sat down with my head in my hands. Before I could have a thought, or erase the one I'd just had, the curtain separating the two halves of the room flew open and there stood an older woman, sixty or seventy years old, no more than five feet tall, with blazing neon red hair. Her eyes were wild with excitement, her tiny, ravaged features stretched to the outer limits of enthusiastic openness.

"Oh, look, Joel, look," she said. She spoke his name using two syllables, as if to rhyme it with the popular Christmas greeting. "Jo-el, look! A new neighbor!"

The woman was looking at me, but she was talking to a man who lay in the other bed staring straight ahead at the wall. He was a deep ash color, about twenty years younger than the woman, with a dark blue, knit ski cap pulled down over his head and forehead as low as it could go without covering his eyes. He held a can of Dr Pepper in his left hand. He wasn't moving at all.

"Oh, dear. Oh, dear, so young," the lady said. "Tsk, tsk, tsk. Look, Jo-el, look. So young."

Joel stared at the wall straight ahead.

"What? What is it, sweetheart?" she asked me. Her tone was softer now, intimate and sympathetic. "Why? Why are you here?"

I stared at her like the Puerto Rican woman had stared at me. Was she real? I thought. Am I really here? Is this really me?

"I've got leukemia."

"Ohh. That's *wunnn*derful," she said. "No, no. Really. If you're gonna have one, that's the best one to have. Right, Jo-el?" She looked over at him for the first time. Joel stared straight ahead.

"*JO-EL!*" she screamed. I nearly leapt up from the bed.

Joel spoke. His voice was weak and gravelly. It seemed as if it were being sent a long distance by an old man trapped deep, deep within. He sounded a lot like the confused character Jim Ignatowski from the TV show *Taxi*.

"Evelynn?" he called.

"She's gone, Jo-el."

"Evelynn??"

"She's gone!"

"Give me a kiss. Evelynn . . . ?"

I got the feeling that this had been going on for a while before I came in.

"Just a . . . little kiss? Evelynn?"

"Why are you being so funny today Jo-el?" his mother asked him. She raised her voice and tried again. "Are you trying to be funny?"

The woman turned back to me. "He's just trying to be funny." Then, shrugging her shoulders, "They think he has a brain tumor, but they can't find it."

"Evelynn? Thirsty . . ."

"There's a Dr Pepper in your hand, Jo-el! Stop being funny!" And she sat down in a chair next to his bed and started reading a magazine, as if she had never spoken to me at all, had never even seen me come in the room.

The only sound for the next several minutes was Joel drinking. Sighing. Gasping. Slurping. Like a man who's been lost in the desert, who is dying of thirst, and who finds a small cup of water. Not nearly enough to survive, but good for one last taste. To be relished and savored for the precious moment's pleasure, and nothing more.

The rest of that weekend was spent having a party. That's what it turned into, in a way. Sometime that Saturday the phone in the room was turned on, and it started ringing and didn't stop. It seemed that everyone I'd ever known or met was calling on the phone.

As soon as the situation had become clear the day before, I had asked Jackie to tell some of our friends. I'd called Lowell and Lillian and a few of my closest friends myself, but each telling of the story took a high toll. My heart would pound as we meandered through the meaningless chatter that begins most conversations. Then I would drop the bombshell and suddenly I'd have a victim on my hands myself. Who could be expected to know how to deal with information like that? These people, my friends, had no better idea than I did what "leukemia" meant. If it meant anything at all to them, the definition would have come from sentimental films on television whose message was: "If you're the strongest, bravest, most loved person to ever walk the Earth, then you will put up a gallant, inspiring fight that will not be quite good enough." That was the only image in my mind.

So Jackie had been putting out calls, helping our friends through their shock, and then I'd quiz her as to every aspect of their reactions. It was somehow titillating. I'd guess that we've all spent *some* time imagining ourselves as the victim of a tragic fate, and wondering just how our loved ones might grieve or rush to our sides. Well, I have. And here it was happening. I was getting a glimpse at my own life from an angle that made me dizzy. Not quite being at my own funeral, but close enough. I was aware of the perversity of these thoughts as I was having them, but I've never had the experience of any kind of awareness diminishing a perversion.

The breadth of the response to my situation stunned me. The room became stuffed with people and balloons as visitors started pouring in through the door. Friends and relatives, friends of my parents and Jackie's relatives — all joined in a macabre reunion. Part celebration of their love for me and part somber disaster scene. After all, there was nothing wrong with me yet. Other than having a deadly disease. I wasn't bedridden. I didn't appear to be or feel terribly ill. I was surrounded by all the people closest to me; every fifteen minutes brought through the door someone dearly loved, whom I'd not seen in months or years; gifts and bouquets were stacked to the ceiling. I was fully dressed, in a state of deep shock, and I was receiving the kind of unconditional love and attention that I'd always dreamed about. I just happened to be sitting in a hospital room with a voice calling "Help me . . ." from down the hall. Things were shockingly festive, broken every so often by a visit from a nurse's aide, who would take my pulse and temperature. I felt like they were embarrassing me at my birthday party.

The way that I had found out about the leukemia in the first place, the reason I had seen Dr. Nixon the Friday before, was that the platelet count in my blood was low. Very low. I didn't know what a platelet was until I met Dr. Scott Kessler a few days before that. Kessler is an ear, nose, and throat specialist who treats a lot of performers — actors and opera singers, dancers and rock stars. He was the doctor who examined Madonna in her film *Truth or Dare* while Warren Beatty squirmed in the background, asking her, "Isn't anything private to you?"

I had gone to see Kessler because I had the flu. Or else something like the flu. Whenever I'm sick, I say I've got the flu. But I wasn't getting better and, as an understudy in *Biloxi Blues,* a Neil Simon play on Broadway, I was scheduled to go on in a few days. The actor who was playing the role of Epstein had decided to take off Yom Kippur, the Jewish holiday. (Neil Simon plays always get interesting around the Jewish holidays. The conflict of loyalties between God and the producer — who's also a Jew. So you feel like you're in trouble with someone whatever you decide to do. But the question is, Who comes to a Neil Simon play on Yom Kippur? And will they even get it? It turns out, who comes are the families of all the Jewish actors who are performing for the Jewish guys taking the day off.)

This Dr. Kessler was extremely thorough. In fact, I probably owe my life to his careful exam and his probing questions. He thought I looked a little pale and asked if I had been bleeding with unusual ease or frequency. I was only there about my sore throat, but since he'd asked, I told him I had a rash that I couldn't explain on my ankles and waist. Dozens of tiny, red pin spots within perfectly smooth skin. Kessler was soon on the floor, kneeling down by my ankles, and I was talking to the top of his head. As he brushed his fingers lightly over my flesh, I talked on and on, telling him that my girlfriend and I had decided it must be heat rash; that I'd had it for about three weeks; asking if he thought I needed any antibiotics for my throat. I think that's the first time I ever felt scared in a doctor's office. Because the doctor seemed concerned, about something in particular, and was finding evidence of what he was concerned about. Dread is what I really felt. A sudden, short, deep stab of dread.

"So, uh, what are you thinking?" I asked him.

Kessler spoke to my foot. "Well," he said, "I think I'd like to take a piece of skin from the back of your throat. I see some of these same red spots there, and we might as well send it off and find out exactly what's going on. I'd also like to send you to the lab and run some blood work."

AIDS. I thought, Holy shit, holy shit, I've got AIDS. He wants to biopsy these red spots because he thinks I've got Kaposi's sarcoma. This was all happening about two months after Rock Hudson's illness became public, so AIDS had finally hit the front pages, so to speak, and was floating in the front of everyone's mind, no matter how small a risk group they were in. As a heterosexual man who struggles to believe in the world as a safe place, the actual danger of AIDS to me personally has zoomed in and out of the foreground over the years. Sometimes I'll be able to convince myself that the danger is extremely remote. Other times, such as when public icons like Rock Hudson and Magic Johnson fall prey, I'll be concerned and feel very vulnerable.

And I read the "Science Times." I have to admit that even before I was ill, I would read the science section of the *New York Times* every Tuesday, trying to match whatever symptoms I might have ever had in my life to whatever diseases happened to be described that week. And I had gotten pretty good at it, too. It's like the crossword puzzle. Just keep doing it and somehow you get better. I was able to give myself a pretty good scare on a regular basis with the science section of the *New York Times.* I had already thought of AIDS.

Dr. Kessler was quickly preparing a small hypodermic needle with an anesthetic, which he then stuck deep into my mouth as I tried not to pass out or punch him and scream for help. He stuck the needle into the soft flesh all the way at the back of my throat. If you opened your mouth really wide and someone shot you with a water pistol from right in front of you, where the water would hit, that's where the needle went. He then picked up an instrument that he gripped like a pair of scissors, but whose gleaming, curved blades faced front. Each time Dr. Kessler distractedly snipped the air, the grinning blades snapped at me like a hungry set of teeth. When he used this tool to clip off a small chunk of meat, Kessler had some trouble. He pulled his hand back, trying to remove his specimen before the blades had finished making their cut. For a moment, it was as if I was being led around the examination room by a miniature hedge clipper stuck down my throat. When he was done I was sent to a blood lab downtown and then went home to wait a couple of days for results.

The next morning the phone rang. It was Dr. Kessler. There were some abnormalities in the test results and he'd like to repeat them.

"Oh? What kind of abnormalities?" I asked him.

And that's how I first learned about platelets. Platelets are an indispensable component of the blood. Tiny disc-shaped cells that help the blood to clot, without which survival would be impossible. Normal level: two hundred thousand to four hundred thousand. For some reason my platelet count was only seventy-five thousand. So the test was repeated. The result, twenty-four hours after the first test, was a platelet count of thirty-five thousand. Less than half the level of the day before. I hadn't even known what was going on inside my body when it was working right. What the fuck was going on inside there now?

This was the beginning of my medical education. The very beginning. Kessler told me that I should see a hematologist, a blood specialist, as soon as possible. The reason for the platelet problem

17

had to be found. I was also told at this point that I was slightly anemic, meaning that I also had a shortage of red blood cells floating around, and that although the level of white blood cells was normal, there seemed to be some abnormally formed ones that needed explaining. None of this meant very much to me because I didn't have any idea what any of these cells did anyway.

When I look back on those conversations with Kessler I'm struck by a feeling of wonder. They were like the last moments of some previous life. When terms and substances that were about to become the focus of my life, the focus of the struggle to keep my life, seemed like a foreign language that I didn't need to learn. As long as I could get by, make my way through with enough knowledge to order from the menu and find the bathroom, I'd be home soon. Back in my own country, where everything was familiar and I knew what to expect and I could feel safe. But I never made it back.

Dr. Zweig arrived in my hospital room sometime Monday morning dressed in a long white coat with the word "Attending" stitched over his heart. He was a tall man, with a bit of a paunch, who sported enormous sideburns and who seemed to be terribly uncomfortable being around someone whom he had been told was ill. He looked just like a giant Groucho Marx. Zweig was followed by another doctor whose name tag read "Fun," and whose eyes remained available for contact just as steadily as Zweig's didn't. Fun didn't speak, he just nodded and smiled.

The only other meeting I'd had with Zweig had been on the phone three days before. He'd returned our call while we were trying to decide what hospital to put me into. At that time he'd said, "I've spoken with the doctor who made the diagnosis and everything seems to be in order. So have a good weekend, and we'll get started by having you admitted on Monday."

"Do we have to wait until Monday?" I asked. "I'd like to get started as soon as possible."

"We only admit emergencies on weekends," he said.

"Acute leukemia's not an emergency?" I heard my voice speaking the words, and I realized right away I might have sounded sarcastic. I was *being* sarcastic. I *meant* to be sarcastic. But, for some reason, I didn't want my new doctor to know that I was capable of sarcasm.

I told him that I was worried about the platelets. I had been told that patients with platelet counts below fifty thousand should be hospitalized. He said that yes, most hospitals would admit me as an emergency case immediately. "But we do things differently here. Don't worry. Have a pleasant weekend. Come to the emergency room if you start bleeding."

"Come in if I start bleeding."

"Yes, that's right." And he was gone.

I hung up the phone and I lost it again. I cried silently at first, and then, with mounting fury, I began to sob so hard, with such intensity, that the sounds that I made became beastly, animalistic. I remember having at least a fleeting sense of embarrassment about it. Not really embarrassment; it's just that my ego didn't completely disappear. It couldn't compete, but it was there. And I didn't like my girlfriend seeing me that way. It didn't fit in with who I had been with her for the past year. I was a strong, successful guy. My career was about to take off.

Well, we all got used to it. It was going to become a constant companion. There would be Evan, and his crying jags. It became commonplace for me to just start crying at various times during the day. The progression was something along the lines of constant, to common, to predictable, to boring, and ultimately, meaningless. Just something that had to be done every day. Like eating, or moving my bowels. An activity that had always had powerful emotional connotations took on the appearance and impact of an involuntary bodily function. Eventually I wouldn't even interrupt whatever I was doing. I would just carry on, while weeping quietly for as long as it needed to last.

My mother had the idea that a Valium might calm me down. I was eager to pop a pill, but we weren't sure if it was safe, so my father, who had been given Dr. Zweig's home phone number before I had spoken to him, put in a call to the doctor.

My dad is a pretty cool dude. I mean, I think he's actually every bit as hyped up and neurotic as I am, he's boiling inside, but he has the ability — a real talent it is, too — to put on a very suave, smooth exterior. It probably comes from running an advertising agency for so many years through so many near crashes. I have vivid memories of seeing him in his office when I was a kid. His feet up on the desk, a phone receiver cradled between his neck and shoulder, huge amounts of tension, concern, and frustration on his face, and a voice being sent through the phone line that was nothing but calm and soothing.

My father spoke into the phone. "Good evening, doctor. Murry Handler calling you. We spoke earlier about my son Evan." My father continued with the question about the Valium and then suddenly stopped talking. I watched his face go through a wide assortment of silent expressions. Finally, he flushed a deep red, as if he were coming to grips with a difficult decision, and said, "All right. Thank you, doctor." And my dad's voice still had that smooth tone, but it was stretched so tight and thin that it seemed about to snap like a rubber band.

"You can take the Valium," was all he said to us.

"What happened?" we all asked. "What was that all about?"

"He told me I was abusing the privilege of having his home phone number," my father said. And he looked like a frightened, scolded schoolboy, in the body of a suddenly old man.

So here was Dr. Zweig, in the flesh. In spite of his dismissal of our concerns, and his assurance that "nothing happens in the hospital over the weekend," we'd managed to get me admitted to Sloan-Kettering first thing Saturday morning. Besides learning that he'd been right about the lethargic pace of weekend hospital life, I found out that news travels fast in the medical gossip network. At our first face-to-face meeting on Monday, Zweig already seemed to know that I had been forced to leave a Broadway show in order to check into the hospital.

"So, you're an actor, huh?" Zweig said it while he stared at his feet and kicked an old, stained piece of gauze bandage along the floor and under the bed.

Before I could answer he said, "I don't really care for Neil Simon plays, myself."

Then he dropped a heavy packet of pages on the meal table next to my breakfast. He took a deep breath, and while he scanned the room with his eyes and touched and studied the cards and gifts left with me over the weekend, he said, "You'll be part of a randomized study. A computer has already selected a new, experimental treatment protocol for you. Half the patients on the study get the new protocol, the other half get the standard protocol. If you agree to be part of the study, you'll have to sign the informed-consent form I just gave you. If you don't sign it, then you'll automatically get the standard protocol." He took a pen from his shirt pocket, laid it on top of the pages he'd thrown down before, and he stood still and looked at me for the first time.

I was sure he was going to have more to say, but it turned out that he was done, so there was a very long pause. Finally he said, "Feel free to read it, if you want."

"Uh, yeah. I think I would like to read it."

"Well, of course you can read it. We want you to read it." With that, Dr. Zweig flopped down into a chair, crushing a large, flat gift box beneath him. He sighed deeply and, staring at the ceiling, he said, "We can't get started until you sign it, though."

Then he again started picking up some of the get well cards. Opening and closing them, running his fingers over them to feel their textures. It was as if they were peculiar artifacts from some ancient civilization whose customs he just couldn't come to understand. His brow would wrinkle up, and he'd let out a sharp breath of air from his nose. Like a disdainful snort. I found myself surprised when he put a card back down without sniffing it and licking it.

Instead, he shot up out of the chair and said, "We'll stop back a little later to pick it up." He turned, and he walked out of the room — leaving Dr. Fun — who nodded and smiled, and then left the room himself.

Jackie now came over and sat next to me on the bed, with her chin resting on my shoulder, and we read through the pages together. We sat in the room by ourselves, side by side, and we learned that I would be treated with massive doses of chemotherapy drugs three times, covering a span of six months. I would spend three of those months in the hospital, most likely being quite ill and in constant danger. A month off to recover would be given between each of the treatments. A successful first remission could be expected in 65 percent of the patients treated this way. Twenty-five percent never achieve remission and die from the leukemia. One out of every ten dies from complications of the treatment itself. The authors of the consent form had an interesting way of describing those people. They wrote of the "patients failing the protocol," rather than the other way around.

The information went on. Let's say you got to be one of the lucky 65 percent. Eighty percent of them have a recurrence of the disease within two years. A second remission is achieved in no more than 50 percent of those cases, and the length of that remission averages in at only one-half the length of a first remission. Third remissions are achieved in less than 5 percent of those who try. This section of the consent form ended with a sentence that was, visually, indistinguishable from those around it. "Survival rates beyond five years do not exceed twenty-five percent."

I looked at that sentence for a long time. I studied the way the ink stained the clean white paper to form the letters, and how the letters formed the words that were conspiring to end my life. I started to cry, and Jackie sat holding me, rubbing my back with the palm of her left hand. Then she cried, too.

I have never felt love for a woman with such a startling intensity as in those moments with Jackie. I'm just like a lot of the men and women that I know. I can't resist someone in direct proportion to how unavailable they are to me. Love, in my life, has been an endless cycle of passionately wooing women to win their love, followed by a scramble to escape as soon as the mission is accomplished. If the escape is successful, they're wooed back with greater and greater cunning and desperation as the drama is played out again and again and again. The repetitions are limited only by each woman's patience, or, more accurately, her endurance. It's not that I don't love them, I do. Every one of them. It's just that I need to feel that I'm about to lose someone to stay interested. So I can win her back. And what's a better way to know you're going to lose your woman than to learn you're about to die? I fell madly in love.

INITIATION

"Do you think you're going to die of leukemia, Evan?"

It was midnight, my third night in the hospital, and Karen was in a chair pulled close next to my bed. With dark hair framing her doughy face in the light leaking in from the hallway, her head seemed to float in space, making her disembodied whisper all the more eerie. Karen was a nurse on her first break after coming on duty at seven, and she'd promised to stop by to talk with me when she got a chance. This wasn't quite the conversation I had been expecting.

"Well, you might," she said. "A lot of people do, you know. Most who get it, in fact. And there's no point in spending all your energy trying to deny it."

Karen and I had met just a few hours earlier, after I had been told by three or four nurses that I really ought to meet her. "Oh, you and Karen would really get along," they all said.

Maybe they were trying to get back at me, I thought. I had already spent the weekend chafing at fitting myself into the "system" of the hospital, and I thought I felt the nurses losing patience with me. But their system seemed nuts. I was constantly being sent for tests with no warning or information provided to me. A nurse would simply arrive in the room and announce that they were "ready for me."

"They're ready for you at X ray!" they'd sing from my doorway. "Ready for you at nuclear medicine!! Ready for you at sonogram!!!" And I was expected to go. If I asked why a test was needed, I was told that it was needed because they wouldn't treat me without it.

These tests happened in far-off branches of the hospital, reached through long underground tunnels. I'd be met in the hallway near the nurses' station by an "escort," without whom I was forbidden to travel off the floor. I would be forced to sit in a wheelchair and be pushed by the escort to wherever it was that they were "ready for me." My first thought was that I'd never again be able to fantasize over the late-night cable television porn ads. I found myself imagining calling one of those escort services and winding up with a wrinkled, old Filipino man pushing a wheelchair ringing my doorbell.

Down in the basement of the hospital, I'd be met by a technician dressed in blue surgical scrubs, giant blue booties, and a blue shower cap. On my very first trip down, a tiny, fast-talking Korean woman pulled me up out of the wheelchair by the sleeve of my shirt. She dragged me through a small, brightly lit waiting room, past rows of patients who were all dressed in their own blue space outfits. These patients were sitting on hard plastic chairs, and they were each staring at the single white floor tile right in front of their own giant blue feet.

The technician pointed me toward a doorway off this room, and, in the most staccato display of human behavior I'd ever seen, she barked at me ferociously. "You go in this room *here!* You take off all your clothes! You take off all your underwears, too! You put on this robe *here!* You come back outside this room!"

I stood still, staring at her dumbfounded.

"*You come back outside this room!* You sit down in this chair *here!*"

The most amazing thing about this scene was that none of the blue patient people even looked up. No, they all kept staring at the floor right in front of their feet. I was afraid that if I put on those blue clothes, I'd become just like them. I wondered if anyone had ever rebelled. I mean, John Wayne had cancer. Did he put up with this?

Then there were the patients back up on the twelfth floor. The screamers, the limbless, the ghostly. My first roommate, Joel, and his mother. Until early Monday morning — when his bed was wheeled out and he inexplicably disappeared, never to be seen again — I'd sat in the room with my family and friends and heard his doctors brusquely charge into the room for their daily visits. On the far side of the curtain they would gruffly lay out absolutely horrifying scenarios and treatment plans in very complex language, then leave and joke and laugh their way down the hall. That was the only thing that stopped Joel and Mom's crazy chatter. After the doctors left they sat in complete silence for ten or fifteen minutes. Mom would then start a one-sided discourse completely twisting and respinning the doctor's report until it was nothing but a fairy-tale version filled with her own fantastic dreams and distortions. If she ever raised any questions about Joel with the doctors or tried to participate in any of the decision making at all she was trampled. Bulldozed by technical terminology and patronizing platitudes until she shut up. Then the doctors would get out of the room fast.

About two-thirds of the other patients I'd seen so far were attached to IV poles whose wheels didn't work. They didn't roll right. I'd watch people, up and down the hall, wrestling with these poles, or coasting out of control until they slammed into the wall. Some of the people had just picked the whole contraption up and were carrying it around with them. But I didn't see anyone fighting back. The few tentative protests that I had made so far, about being pushed in a wheelchair, say, were met by the nurses with chuckles and nods to each other that seemed to say, "Oh, how cute. One of those. We haven't seen one in a long time." Always clear in their communication was that they knew exactly how to deal with my kind.

Just that morning, two nurses had come into my room to make the bed. They were being really friendly, asking me to tell them all about myself. "Oh! An actor. How nice," one of them said. "We've had a lot of actors here."

And the other one said, "Sure, sure. Johnny Cazale died on this floor."

So maybe Karen was my punishment. Sent to torment me into submission and cooperation. She cooed spookily into the darkness. "Are you religious, Evan?" she asked. "Maybe you'd better spend some time thinking ... about *faith.*"

Sometime later that night, I don't know how long after I'd fallen asleep, I was startled awake by my new roommate, Robert, crying out. His voice sounded like it was coming from the bottom of his soul. He said, "Hi ...," with a combination of wonder and joy and resigned acceptance. Inevitability, that's what I heard him express. And it was terrifying.

My immediate thought was that he was dreaming about meeting someone he had never expected to see again, and that he was being torn away from them at the same instant as the reunion was taking place. And "hi ..." was all that he managed to get out before they were gone. Then I thought it sounded as if he might be meeting God. And that was the next thing he said: "God!" I put the pillow over my head. I wondered how a person might *create* faith in their heart. Was it possible? Could a person *will* himself to believe in God? To entrust his safety to a universe that had landed him in this situation to begin with?

Earlier that morning I'd received my first mail at the hospital. One of the cards was from a friend of my parents, a woman who had adopted fundamentalist Christianity several years before, after her oldest son was diagnosed as schizophrenic. The card had a colorful painting of Jesus Christ on the front. His expression was warm and friendly, his arms spread open with his palms facing upward in a welcoming gesture. I opened the card, and the printed message said "Only when you accept Jesus Christ as your savior will your soul be safe in the kingdom of Heaven." I closed the card fast. I felt like I'd just received a letter threatening my life. From a close family friend. Or was it being threatened by Jesus Christ himself?

I was really shaken by that card, until I opened the one from my parents' neighbors. A couple whom I used to baby-sit for, and whom I still saw a few times every year. Theirs was one of those pop-up cards — when I opened it, a picture of a bouquet of flowers unfolded toward me. They had written their message in pen down the side. "Dear Evan," it said. "We want you to know we are thinking of you, and we will always remember you." We all had a good laugh over that one. And it made me forget about Jesus threatening my life. For a while.

I began giving more and more thought to what I might depend on to pull me through the months ahead. I realized that, in my nonreligious family, the only faith that had ever been instilled in me, during my childhood, was a faith in myself. Even if I had wanted to respond to Jesus' offer of salvation, it seemed impossible to impose an entirely new set of beliefs on such short notice. But I began to think that if I could find some form of spirituality that relied primarily on me, and on maximizing my own potential, maybe I'd have a shot. I had no idea what form it should take or where it would come from. But, in the hopes that pleas from even the most skeptical souls can be heard in Heaven, I started praying to whatever God might be willing to listen.

*　　*　　*

I'd been hearing for days about the "chemo nurses," how great they were, what good hands I'd be in. I couldn't understand why special nurses were needed for the chemotherapy, though. I'd been having my veins punctured for four days already. To leak blood out, to pour liquids in. Some of the vampires were definitely better than others, but why "chemo nurses"?

These women wore special little caps, like what you'd expect to see on nurses in a 1950s movie. They acted pert and spunky, wore their hair in Donna Reed flips, and, in so doing, they almost succeeded in disguising the grave seriousness they brought to the task of correctly identifying the live body in front of them.

One of the team of two took hold of my left wrist with one of her hands. Her other hand gripped my fingers, and, with me effectively immobilized, she positioned the hospital name tag bracelet in front of her face and read my forearm like it was a fortune cookie.

"What is your name?" she asked.

After I told her, the other nurse said, "Now spell it."

This was not Donna Reed anymore. Thinking that they were through with my limb, I sent a message from my brain to what had been my arm to go quietly back by my side. But my arm no longer belonged to me. The chemo nurse held tight and seemed to notice not one bit that I had tried, with a good deal of strength, to reclaim it. She then proceeded to repeat my name herself, repeat the spelling of my name, and read off the patient ID number to her partner, who was checking the information off on pink sheets of paper attached to a clipboard. When I again thought that they were through, the nurses suddenly switched roles, and the one with the clipboard began barking out all the facts over again as the one who held my wrist studied the ID bracelet, mouthing the words silently as she read along.

When the security check was complete the two women *popped*, like a bubble bursting, back into the Betty Crocker mode. They were asking me about my life, gurgling and fawning over everything I said, as they quickly, gracefully, with military precision, attached tubing and clamps to the IV line already in my arm. They had a system wherein one of them spoke with me, distracted me, while the other performed the intricate mechanical maneuvers. I had the thought that this must be how animals feel, in the moments before they are expertly slaughtered, never having quite enough time to figure out what it is that's being done to them.

My mother and father were in the room with me. We were all extremely apprehensive about the procedure about to take place. On one hand, it was a very welcome event to be getting started in the treatment of the leukemia. On the other hand, we were quivering in nervous anticipation of all the worst side effects that might be right around the corner. We could have guessed about the nausea and the vomiting that would follow. No one had to tell me that my hair would fall out. But what we'd learned about the mechanics of the treatment itself was a frightening shock to all of us.

The chemotherapy agents would be administered over four consecutive days. These drugs, one of them called Ara-C (not a bad name for a sports drink, I thought), and the other 4-DMDR (a character from the *Star Wars* trilogy?), would severely damage my bone marrow and all blood-making capabilities, wiping out most of my immune system. For that reason, it was expected that I would almost certainly become extremely ill, fairly quickly, with an infection caused by whatever organism got to me first. At that time the doctors would try to make an accurate diagnosis and administer antibiotics before the infections overwhelmed my organs.

Less serious, but more immediately on our minds, was the nurses' repeated caution to *immediately* tell them if I experienced any burning or tingling sensations while the drugs were being given. This was thanks to Dr. Zweig's imposing recommendation, delivered as an already-made decision, that it would be best for me to receive my chemotherapy, all transfusions, all medications, all electrolyte infusions, through single IV lines inserted into veins in my arms. These lines were plugged in using needles, by IV nurses who made regular rounds, and lasted no more than two or three days before they had to be replaced with a new needle. These same lines were used to draw blood, though not very effectively. Trying to draw blood from one of these peripheral lines often caused a blowout of the vein, which then required a fresh stabbing to draw blood, as well as another puncture to get a new IV line going.

The alternative to this was to have a Broviac catheter implanted into my chest. This was a permanent tube, one end of which would be inserted into a vein in my neck. The other end of the tube would then be tunneled under my skin until it poked out a small hole in the chest area. The tube then branched off into two smaller ones, and, with two little rubber ports plugged on the ends for sticking the needles into, no more stabbings! Almost all the patients on the floor had these access lines in, and seemed relieved to have them. They and the nurses gave me odd glances when I said that I was going to have my chemo on my arms alone, but Dr. Zweig told me that there would be no problem, that those access lines could get infected, and why increase the risk? Not yet knowing the unusual level of discomfort this portended, even within the harsh context of chemotherapy treatment, I consented to be treated with a minimum of risk and with a maximum of pain.

So, as the chemo nurses placed a metal carrying case on the bed next to me, and as they opened it and withdrew a large, clear plastic cylinder containing a bright orange liquid that was to be injected into a vein in my left arm — specifically my left arm, because I'm right-handed — our fears were of the burning or tingling sensations that I might feel as the chemical was pushed into my veins and into my body. This chemical, if administered *very* slowly, *very* carefully, over the course of fifteen minutes for this one tube alone, could glide into the vein and cause only the predictable damage in the expected areas of the body. But if pushed into the vein too quickly, if any leaked out of the vein, or, God forbid, if the needle slipped out of the vein, the chemical would burn and blister the flesh, causing intense pain for months, and leaving permanent scars. As one of the hipper male IV nurses, who'd been around to witness it, had told me, "That shit would tear your ass up."

Jackie had already apologized for her squeamishness and left the room, so it was just me and Mom and Dad. I was terrified, and I think my mother was more so. But, bless her heart, she was staying in the room with me. I knew she wanted to run and hide, that she would have given almost anything to get out of that room. And at any other time in my life I would have lost my temper. I would have scolded her and told her to go ahead and leave if she couldn't hide her agony. But on that day I just wanted her help. Any help she could muster. My mother, trembling and close to tears, was holding my free hand and whispering encouragement to me, as the container of orange chemical was solidly clicked and locked into place at the end of the tube that was connected to the needle that was in my arm.

And that's when the chemo nurse said it.

"You've been to the sperm bank, right, Evan?"

I said, "... Huh?"

The two nurses turned toward each other in what looked like a perfectly choreographed move. They gave a priceless, puzzled glance, and then turned, again in unison, back to me.

The other one spoke. She addressed me slowly, drawing out each syllable, as if I suffered from the most severe of mental disabilities. "Evan, didn't your doctor tell you about the *sperm bank?*"

I answered her with the same controlled exasperation. "No. No, he didn't. Is there something I need to know about the *sperm bank?*"

This time they didn't look at each other. With the swiftness and urgency of a bomb squad team they clicked and pulled and had the orange cylinder detached from my arm. The cylinder went back into the metal carrying case labeled "Biohazard," the two picnic basket–type lids were slammed shut, and the box was picked up off the bed and placed on a table several feet away.

"We'll be right back," one of the nurses said, and they turned and left the room. A split second later the other one reappeared, grabbed the biohazardous metal picnic basket, and fled once again.

My mother was still holding my hand.

And so I was welcomed into the wild and wacky world of sperm-banking. I was issued a pass that allowed me to leave the hospital. Insurance regulations had prohibited my leaving the hospital at all until now, under the assumption that anyone well enough to go outside and breathe fresh air is not sick enough to necessitate payment for a hospital room. That's a rule that continued through all my hospitalizations in New York. No matter how beneficial the sunshine might have been, how therapeutic a walk around the block might have seemed, the only place to be outdoors was on a ten-foot-wide terrace on the fifteenth floor of a building holding eighteen floors of people.

Jackie and I left the hospital, and we headed for the sperm bank — on Madison Avenue. Nothing but the best address for my progeny. Along the way we had our first taste of the disturbing realization that everything in the world was just as it had been five days ago. New York City, and certainly the world beyond, didn't seem to have any interest in the devastation that we were in the midst of, or any awareness at all of the teeming, seething society inside the building that we had just left. We started joking about the absurdity of walking around the streets of Manhattan with a deadly disease and played with the idea of going to the airport and getting on a plane. Paris, perhaps. Definitely Europe, somewhere. Maybe if we went someplace where we were unknown, where there was no history, then the whole situation would vanish along with our old identities.

I also had the first notion of the depth of trust that I was being forced to give to an entire community of strangers. State-certified as they might be, those doctors and nurses and pharmacists and technicians, they were still unknown to me. And this was my life on the line. My existence. My confidence in them was a suspicious one at best, and my confidence in the state that regulated them was somewhat lower than that.

Call it denial, and I guess that's what it was, but as we reached the IDANT Andrology Laboratories on Madison Avenue I had the additional thought that it was at least *possible* that I didn't have anything seriously wrong with me at all. Maybe no one inside Sloan-Kettering really had a disease. How many of them had been shown the slides of their abnormal tissues? Shown the slides, been taught how to understand them, how to compare them to normal tissues, and been satisfied enough to allow strangers to carve them up or administer lethal doses of toxic chemicals? I hadn't. What if this was the way that the medical establishment, the government, did its research? Its experimentation. Take every forty or fiftieth person who walks in the door, tell them they have a dread disease, and get them into the laboratory, the torture chamber, of their own free will. For their own benefit. I'd read news accounts of governments doing things just as diabolical in the past. My paranoia felt not only justified to me, but wise. Maybe we were all just being good little citizens and doing as we were told. Just remove your jewelry, drop your clothes in the bin, and have a nice hot shower before we assign you a bunk.

At IDANT I was given a clipboard by a woman dressed in white standing behind a window. There were forms to be filled out before I could open my bank account. I didn't realize I was staring into space until I heard Jackie say, "Sweetie? Sweetie, are you all right?"

I looked up at her, and with my IDANT-supplied pencil poised, I asked, "How do you spell 'leukemia'?"

Jackie spelled the word for me, slowly, and then I said, "I'm sorry this is happening to you."

Back at the window, the woman in white handed me a small plastic container with a lid. She told me that I was to go into room number three, "produce" a specimen, and, without touching the inside of the container or contaminating the specimen in any way, "deposit" it in the cup, and bring it back to the window. She then gave me a key on a ring with a large plastic "3" attached to it, handed me a thick manila folder, and called, "Next!"

I was tempted to ask her *how* I was supposed to "produce" the specimen, but I resisted, and the question that I didn't really need to ask was answered when I got inside room number three. After struggling with the giant key chain I opened the door, and I was met with a gust of *freezing* cold air. Inside the tiny refrigerated room was a simple metal folding chair, a miniature three-legged side table, and a box of tissues. I sat down in the chair and put the manila folder on my lap. I must have been terribly unsophisticated in the ways of sperm-banking, but I had no idea what I had been given in the folder. When I opened it and found about a dozen pornographic magazines, I was stunned. Then I giggled.

Did they subscribe, I wondered? Or was it someone's job to go shopping periodically, to keep the supply varied and up-to-date?

I was really interested in checking out the magazines. I like pornography, I find it fascinating. And not that it doesn't turn me on, it does. But in addition to that, I'm always astonished by the idea of people making really hard-core pornography. Who they are, what it was like there at the time, how it felt to them. And there was some really hard-core stuff in there. All mixed in with the *Playboy* and the *Oui*. There were the *Juggs*, the *Beaver*, the *Ass Fuckers*.

I was actually a little bit thrilled with the magazines in my lap. I still haven't gotten over a certain adolescent relationship to pornography. A kind of substitution fantasy that turns the book, and my feelings toward it, into something very much like those I'd have toward a woman. There have been times that I've stopped not very far short of setting a candlelit dinner table for myself and a magazine. It's probably magnified by the fact that I never got over my inhibitions surrounding buying the stuff or about being open and shameless about my interest in it. Maybe this confession will help. Either that, or six more years of therapy.

And, Jackie was with me. We had decided to try and make sperm-banking fun, and to try not to lose touch with our sex life, by having Jackie help me to jerk off into the cup, inside the refrigerated room, on Madison Avenue. *Very* sexy.

Jackie took off her shirt, and instantly broke out into the most extreme case of goose bumps I had ever seen. As we started to fool around in that room, I wanted nothing more than to be left alone.

Jackie and I had fallen in love quickly, about a year before, in a small town in the Catskill Mountains. How appropriate for two Jews. But this wasn't the Borscht Belt Catskills. Tannersville was a rustic, small town that came alive only during the winter, when the local ski mountain became a prime destination for thousands of New Yorkers.

We met in the summer, when a theater company that we were both involved with held its annual artists' retreat. I had come up as a result of having met a woman named Rachel through mutual friends after one of my last performances in a play called *Found a Peanut*, at Joseph Papp's New York Shakespeare Festival. Rachel and I decided to rent a car and share a ride up to Tannersville.

At least, that's what I thought we'd decided. Upon arriving I found myself immediately infatuated with the slim, wavy-haired, blond woman exercising on the front lawn. Jackie was dressed in dark blue sweat pants that had shrunk enough to show off her still girlish athleticism. I followed her up the steps to the porch, smitten by just the sight of her, and when she turned to face me and I saw her blue eyes smiling at me from her adorably lopsided face, I felt like I'd been away on a trip somewhere and had just returned home. Jackie said "Hello," giggled, and disappeared. For the rest of that afternoon I fantasized about how I might get to speak with her, as I was relentlessly pursued by my driving companion. Unknown to me, as I had parked the car, Rachel had responded to the innkeeper's inquiry as to whether we were a couple requiring a shared room with a simple "not yet."

The tension mounted through the weekend as I maneuvered my way into private walks and talks with Jackie, trying not to insult anyone in the process. I wasn't being coy or rude. While I certainly suspected that Rachel was interested in me, nothing had been spoken.

I felt it would have been presumptuous of me to explain a lack of interest to a woman who hadn't actually communicated any to me yet. At least not in a way that I was capable of understanding at that time in my life. Acknowledging my own attractiveness to a woman who might pursue it aggressively was way beyond my limitations at twenty-three years old.

The climax, or lack of one, came on an oppressively humid night during Mario Cuomo's keynote address to the 1984 Democratic National Convention. I was lying facedown, with no shirt on, in my room of the Forest Inn, with Rachel on a chair facing me. My denial could not have been more complete. Rachel stared at me longingly, offering conversation, and making gallant attempts to rekindle the flirtation that I was able to engage in only while swimming in a large group, as we had been the night we met in Manhattan. I, meanwhile, was straining furiously to hear Cuomo's voice delivering his rousing speech, as it floated across the hall from a small clock radio next to Jackie's bed, where I wanted to be. I listened to that speech as if I was in the room with her. I raised the volume of my comments, my oohs and aahs and groans of appreciation, my *breathing*, all in the attempt to share that night with her, to use Mario and his vision of the future to connect us, and to fuse one of our own, together. Weeks and months later Jackie and I joked that Rachel would have to be invited to our wedding.

Now, in our cozy IDANT cubicle, Jackie was being every bit the ultimate of what someone in my position could hope for. Until my diagnosis, however, our relationship, after one year, had reached a point of stasis, and I had begun to feel dissatisfied. Our lovemaking, up to this point, had been deeply affectionate, but hardly uninhibited, and the frequency had tapered off, at times to the point where I would wonder if Jackie was even still attracted to me. But I was well aware that I was going to need a sturdy support system for what lay ahead, and both my fear of abandonment and Jackie's startling devotion had caused me to reexamine my doubts. When she offered to spice up the sperm-banking expedition I was moved, I was more than happy, even if a little bit self-conscious, and I welcomed her gift. I also didn't feel like I had the right to turn her down. In any case, it became excruciatingly clear to me that I was about to have one of the most intimate sexual encounters of my life, inside a locked closet, with strange men masturbating for medical purposes on either side of me.

Coming into a cup is not easy. I was surprised to learn that, then surprised that I was surprised, because I had surely never tried it before, so how could I know? It's not so much the simple act of hitting a target with an ejaculation, though I'm not sure that's really so simple either, but the repeated instructions ". . . not to touch the inside of the cup, *in any way!*" that posed problems. Especially when combined with the warning that "**the greatest number of sperm are contained in the *first spurt*.**" Who would have known? The woman in white at the window, that's who.

I was lying on my side, on blue industrial carpeting, with my pants around my knees. I was clutching the all-too-small plastic specimen jar in my left hand, holding it close to, *but not touching,* my penis, as I masturbated frantically and felt an orgasm approaching. My mind was soaring, my surroundings spinning in and out of my awareness, as I struggled to give myself over to pleasure in this situation.

After all, orgasms feel good. And that became a problem. I was not having fun, I hated where I was, my reason for being there was catastrophic, and nothing had happened to me over the past week that was not demeaning and humiliating. I was on my last outing from an existence of torture that was about to begin, having my last free moments before a time of great physical pain, and, as my body went rigid and convulsed, I came into the cup, thinking only of the story to be told to my children one day of how they came to be.

My children, who were dripping down the inside of the jar. My children, who were mostly in the first spurt.

I exhaled slowly, deeply. I got my breathing back under control, all the while refusing to grant life to the groan of pleasure and release that was reaching up and out from inside my chest. I had a momentary image flash through me of what it would be like if God became a rapist, and that perhaps that was what He had just done to me.

Back outside room number three there was a line of men, containers in hand, waiting to get to the woman in the window. I was fourth or so from the front, glad to be that far back, because my greatest wish at that moment was that the semen in the cup would cool off before I had to hand it over. Blood, somehow, would be different. Urine, slightly humbling. I had, in the past, handed over stool specimens, still warm in their waxed cardboard containers that so resemble those in which take-out food is packed up, and felt embarrassed. Nothing though, for me, can match the emasculatory glory of standing with four other men; a fresh, hot ejaculate in hand; waiting to hand it over to a stranger; a woman, in uniform; who then proceeds to place the now sealed plastic container on a scale, and weigh it.

That's right, the specimen is handed over, and, in full view of all the others in line, its weight is checked and announced, just like at the weigh-in before a boxing match. The weight is then recorded in a giant, hardcover book, and that is how the fee for storage is determined. I wondered if any of the other men had the same instinctive urge as I did to applaud one another as each weight was announced, to cheer each other in our accomplishment, having produced these massive specimens, as only a man can do. "Weighing in at just under two ounces!"

Instead, we all waited quietly, staring down at the white lids to our tiny plastic jars. Each here for his own secret reason. Each one hoping someday to reach back in time, from a better future, and to thaw out a piece of himself, preserved intact from how he was today.

TRANSFORMATION

There is little chance that I could ever give an accurate, visceral impression of what the chemotherapy treatment for acute leukemia felt like physically. But believe me, if the body had any sense of its own, it would not allow what was about to happen to begin. Death be damned, no body would allow itself to be punctured and poisoned, to be reduced to a state of heinous malfunction without an egocentric personality running the show. The body knows that the universe is just as accepting of its death as of its life. Only the frightened person steering the ship believes that the Earth needs them alive as desperately as they need Her to live.

And that's what makes chemotherapy possible.

Leukemia itself is simply an overabundant production of nonfunctioning white blood cells. Like a switch getting stuck on, these cells continue to divide and reproduce, overcrowding the bone marrow and interfering with the production of other cells. The bone marrow is the birthplace of all the body's blood cells, and so the entire immune system, all nutrition, and all clotting capability are dependent upon its precise functioning. Therefore, if untreated, one would quickly die from a lack of immune response, due to the shortage of healthy white cells; from bleeding, as a result of the lack of platelets (a process that had already begun on my waist and ankles — my "rash" was actually an array of *petechiae*, tiny blood capillaries that were leaking); or from problems stemming from anemia, the shortage of red blood cells, which transport oxygen to all the body's organs. The basic premise behind traditional chemotherapy treatment for leukemia is to kill off as much of the patient's bone marrow as possible without actually killing the patient. This scheme can go wrong in a number of ways.

When chemotherapy drugs are introduced into the body, they destroy the bone marrow, as well as many other cells in the body. The cells that reproduce the fastest consume most of the toxins, thereby offering the possibility that the marrow cells that are out of control will be obliterated before the ones that are behaving appropriately. These variations in absorption speed also explain some of the side effects of the treatment: loss of hair, stomach distress, terrible mouth sores, as the skin lining the mouth and throat dies and peels away. Cells in these areas of the body naturally have a fast metabolic rate, and so also absorb a good deal of the medicine.

The greatest concern, however, is in regard to the bone marrow. There is no perfect way to gauge just how much poison can be tolerated by the marrow, while successfully eradicating the leukemia cells. Too much can result in the same quick death as the leukemia would have provided itself: from infection, bleeding, or anemia. More often, though, there is an extended battle while the patient's blood counts drop down to nothing, and life is preserved through transfusions of red cells and platelets, and infections are fought off with antibiotics and antifungal and antiviral drugs. Since white blood cells constitute a body's immune system, they can't be transfused. The white cells from the donor's body would perceive the recipient's tissues as an invading force and attack them. Eventually, hopefully, the marrow then recovers and resumes its own life support. If, after the marrow's recovery, no abnormal cells can be detected under a microscope, the leukemia is said to be in remission.

This period, between the giving of the drugs and the marrow's regeneration, is the time of pain and horror. Any organism has the capability to overwhelm the body. Infections attack suddenly and can be relentless. The specter of deadly hemorrhaging lurks in every moment. Blood transfusions are therefore essential and unending, and each transfusion requires premedication with powerful drugs and carries risks of its own. Any infection present in the donor's blood, including serious ones like hepatitis, can be passed on to the recipient. This danger zone can easily last three weeks and is spent enduring high fevers, furious full-body rashes, nosebleeds, vomiting, and drug-induced stupors. That's the scenario if everything goes as well as possible. Among the other possibilities are an internal hemorrhage, sepsis of the blood from bacterial infection (leading to organ failure and possibly death), and, one of the great fears, pneumonia.

During this time the patient is referred to by the medical professionals as being "nadir," or, loosely translated, "nothing," due to the zero level of white blood cells in the daily blood count. Colored signs are posted on the patient's door advising all who enter to take "neutrapoenic precautions" to avoid bringing any germs into the room. The "neutrapoenic" patient has no measurable immune function, and so, a surgical mask and plastic gown must be worn by all visitors. Hands must be scrupulously washed before each entry, even though any physical contact is forbidden. The patient is required, in spite of the fevers and the rashes, to shower three times a day with rough sponges soaked in iodine, to avoid fungus growing on the skin. Food must all be either cooked or peeled, as the whole world turns hostile and dangerous, and the body is transformed into nothing more than a defenseless host for myriads of parasitic organisms that had been previously unimagined. Suddenly, it's as if you can feel them walking on your skin; smell them in the air you breathe; taste them in every bite of food. In the strange vernacular of the *Bhagavad Gita,* life is become danger, and each moment survived carries the seed that could grow destruction.

Early on in the treatment my brother, Lowell, came to visit me. My brother, at this time, was my closest friend in life. We had only recently stopped living together in my apartment, we spoke constantly by telephone, and it was rare that one of us got invited anywhere that the other didn't end up going as well. Until about a year before, we even had girlfriends who were also roommates. We would tromp over there together, like two happy puppies, making jokes about getting laid and calling ourselves "The Breast Brothers." We always said that we wished that the women were sisters as well. Then it would be perfect.

Lowell and his Touretticisms could cause quite a commotion when he'd show up at the hospital, so I had tried to limit his visits. The last time he'd come by was a couple of weeks before; since then, as it was designed to, the treatment had destroyed my bone marrow and my immune system, and so I was suffering from a serious infection. That's why I was on "Shake and Bake."

"Shake and Bake" was the nurses' playful name for the drug amphotericin. Amphotericin is a yellow liquid used to fight systemic fungal infections that's administered intravenously over a period of hours each day for two weeks. It causes raging fevers, 104 to 105 degrees, which are then followed by violent, shaking chills. We're talking *Exorcist,* bed-shaking, shaking chills. Whenever the chills came it was important to call a nurse right away so she could give me a shot of Demerol, which, when mixed with the Thorazine and Nembutal that I was already getting for nausea (as well as to control the drug-induced hiccoughs that wracked my body for days on end), would calm the chills, which were then replaced by a raging fever. This was all done to save my life. This was called "Shake and Bake."

I had been shaking and baking for several days already, and, in addition to having lost my hair from the chemotherapy, I had turned the color of a lobster from the amphotericin, the Demerol, the Thorazine, and the Nembutal. I have never seen the color red displayed with such purity as it was by my flesh on "Shake and Bake."

"Hnn. Hnn. Hnn."

I heard my brother doing his Tourettic dance down the hall. He stopped outside the room to read the name card on the door, and I could see half his body, bobbing up and down in the door frame.

Satisfied that he was in the right place he bounced into the room, with his head down, carrying flowers and a wide smile on his face, and he said, "Brother!"

When he looked up and saw me he said, "Oh, shit. Sorry." And he turned and he left the room.

He had already disappeared around the corner by the time I called out to him. I heard him stop at the familiar sound of my voice.

"Evan? Evan? Where are you?"

"Lowell, come back. I'm in the room."

And my brother *slooowly* crept back into the room, staring at me in disbelief, like we were two bad actors trapped in our own version of *The Metamorphosis.* The flowers he held were pointing down at the ground, about to slip out of his hand.

"I . . . I didn't recognize you," he said.

Then we had our visit.

My parents, though they would be enraged whenever I suggested it, were also exhibiting some startling effects from the strain of my diagnosis and hospitalization. They didn't cease to function, but their functioning was thrown off-kilter, and their judgment became confused. My parents seemed cowed by fear in the presence of the doctors and bewildered by any attempt to comprehend the disease and its treatment. I was becoming increasingly enraged by what seemed to be either their inability or refusal to grasp even the most basic facts about leukemia and the process that I was undergoing. The only reason that I even suspected purposeful unwillingness on their part was that my brother had been living with a rare neurological disorder for years — medical terminology was not foreign to any of us. Why had they abruptly lost their ability to process even rudimentary information? The fact was that my parents were in a state of deep shock.

The treatment plan called for me to be hospitalized for a few days to receive the large doses of chemotherapy intravenously. I would then be discharged to wait as most of my blood-making bone marrow (and so, my immune system) died off. As a result of this marrow damage it was expected that I would inevitably develop an infection, which would declare its presence as a fever. At that point it would become urgent to return to the hospital, *without delay,* for emergency treatment, which would last until the bone marrow recovered. The whole process, from beginning to end, would last about a month.

Since it could be anywhere from one to ten days until the drugs did enough damage for the fever to occur, I would be discharged from the hospital to wait. My parents were able to borrow, through phone calls to friends, a spacious Upper East Side apartment, to be used as our "safe house," to bide the time until a fever popped up. However, while they were able to engineer these luxurious accommodations and willing to abandon their own lives while trying to save mine, any input from them into the many critical medical decisions required was consistently frightening due to their lack of understanding of the issues involved. My mother had even tried, the night before the fateful visit to Dr. Nixon, to get me to take a dose of a powerful steroid — albeit at the urging of a misguided, hometown family physician. One possible explanation for the symptoms that had driven me to the doctor was an autoimmune disorder that would have been treated with steroids had that proven to be the case. But in her panic, and with the encouragement of the man we'd long referred to as the "chicken soup doctor," my mother was trying to convince me to treat something that was still undiagnosed, in a manner that could have prevented accurate detection of the leukemia. This kind of well-intentioned, but potentially dangerous, clouded thinking had remained common all through the first hospitalization.

This infuriated me. While I was aware that I was being ruthlessly demanding, no matter how hard I tried to appreciate the trauma they were enduring as parents, I could not transcend my rage and disappointment over the limits of their strength. My wrath grew out of the perception that I was being denied the opportunity to have a collapse of my own. No matter how I might have wanted to put my fate into the hands of others, it was all too clear to me that my existence in the hospital was going to be one of clawing to survive. Forget the glamorous ring of the name of a world-class research institution. The reality was that there were not enough pillows and blankets to go around. Sheets and pillowcases were stained and in shreds. To get enough of these items, as well as towels, required going to other areas of the floor, or to other floors, and swiping them before someone else got there.

There was an even greater shortage of nurses and doctors. I quickly learned that several of the routinely prescribed drugs at the hospital, used as transfusion premedications or to combat dangerous chemotherapy side effects, gave me horrendously adverse reactions. This should not have been such an extraordinary problem, for there were other drugs available to do the same job. The problem was that, to save time, one drug would routinely be ordered for all the patients on the floor undergoing similar treatment. The doctors writing the orders didn't necessarily know my case personally. When the nurses would bring the medication to the room, I would have to point out that, if they'd check my chart, they'd see that I couldn't tolerate that particular drug. This would throw everyone's schedule into chaos.

The doctor would have to return to the floor to write another prescription, and this could take an hour or more; the new prescription would have to be sent to the pharmacist to be filled; but by the time the new drug arrived and could be administered, the time limit for administering the blood would have expired, and so new blood would have to be ordered from the blood bank. I would be confronted, on several occasions, by a red-faced nurse who, overwhelmed by his or her own responsibilities and the lack of resources available to meet them, would scream at me for the problems that I was causing. Since I might very well be barely conscious at the time, it would fall to someone else to keep the nurses from giving me the wrong medicine. Often, the only way to do this was to scream back at them, louder, and for a longer period of time than they could afford to stay and berate me for refusing to take the drugs that would make me ill.

The energy required for hunting for linens or monitoring the nurses' work was something that I couldn't consistently muster. If my parents couldn't remember the names of the drugs that gave me bad reactions, then they couldn't help me in one of the many ways that I needed help. If they couldn't challenge the bullying nurses, then I had to remain eternally alert to do it myself. Luckily, Jackie became quite good at this. "Look, you're not giving him that shit. Just call the fucking doctor and stop wasting so much time!" she'd scream. Finally, they'd leave and do just that.

The next day the doctor would apologize for the mix-up and promise to write clearer orders, and a nurse would stop by my room to tell me, "I hear your girlfriend has a bad attitude. You know, that can affect your care. Why can't you be more like Andy down the hall? He comes around with us and helps us make the beds."

*   *   *

My poor mother and father didn't escape the nurses' wrath either. When they made such heroic gestures as driving an hour into Manhattan during a blizzard, or walking six deserted blocks in the howling winds and flying glass of a full-fledged hurricane — all at my request — to be by my side during procedures that frightened me, they were scolded mercilessly.

"Do you know how many parents get sick while their kids are in the hospital?" the nurses would chide. "Do you know how many parents we have to admit because of heart attacks? Do you know how many die in car accidents?" The message being imparted made complete sense, but the manner of delivery put everyone even more on edge.

In spite of the harsh warnings, or perhaps due to the added stress of them, my mother was given a prescription for Halcion by a doctor not associated with Sloan-Kettering. Halcion was the drug preferred by all the hospitals that I visited for helping the patients to sleep. One didn't need to request it; it was standard issue, handed off at dusk with a collection of other colorful tablets in a tiny paper cup. Halcion is a drug that has been in the news of late. It's been banned in some countries, and there has been at least one movement to remove it from the U.S. market. Many believe there is evidence, available even then, that Halcion may occasionally cause severe depression, mania, and suicidal or homicidal tendencies in anxious individuals. Great stuff to give to people torn out of their lives and thrown into an institution days or hours after learning they have cancer.

My mother was told to take a portion of a pill whenever she felt tense. A few weeks into my first hospitalization she took some before getting on the New Jersey Turnpike for a two-hour drive. Half an hour later she drove off the road and wrecked her car. My father had, himself, taken to drinking tall iced tea glasses filled to the brim with bourbon and water, and, within a week, he also ruined a car in a potentially catastrophic single auto accident. They both vehemently denied that their automobile accidents had anything to do with my illness, and became furious when I suggested that they were crumbling when I needed them most. I began to feel even more alone and cast off from anyone whose sanity I could recognize. I started to think that perhaps I was losing my mind and everyone else was behaving rationally. Jackie was my only connection to anyone who seemed to make sense, and we insulated ourselves with greater and greater determination. This upset my parents even more, as I limited the frequency of their visits, and Jackie and I grew closer together and farther and farther away from everyone else.

Before long, there was little or nothing that my parents could do right in my eyes. Every genuine effort on their part was marred by my lack of tolerance for the smallest slip. If I asked for a Coke and my father brought back orange soda, in my totally dependent condition, this was enough to set me off. On the occasions when they did something truly wonderful, like ordering me a telescope for my birthday, an item I had always wanted, I exploded at them for being overly generous only in the midst of a crisis. I cried and screamed and accused them of trying to comfort me with gifts because they really had no faith that I was going to survive. I greedily took for granted, as my birthright, the sacrifices they were making, in terms of time, money, and emotional investment, and showed them very little gratitude for the hours they spent shopping for my comfort, or for the swarms of people they steered toward the blood bank to make donations for me. I'm not claiming that I was anything other than a holy terror myself.

Rightfully or wrongfully, I was unable to forgive the particular manifestations of my parents' state of shock and the hypervigilance that it necessitated on my part. I craved, I dreamed of a scenario, where I could have broken down myself. Abandoned all sense of responsibility, while feeling safe and well protected from any more danger than I was already in. But that wasn't the situation as I perceived it, and so I learned to fight. I learned that I must always remain in control, double-check everyone's work, and trust no one completely. I must have been sheer hell to be around. But I know that my cantankerousness saved my life on several occasions.

In spite of this tidal wave of hostile bombardment, over the next few weeks I became the most optimistic human being I had ever met. I learned what I would call a kind of "opportunistic optimism." The basis for the transformation was the simple realization that I could, out of sheer will and necessity, alter my beliefs about things. I began to embrace any notions that would enhance my tendencies for hope, while practicing powerful mental techniques to banish any thought patterns that might interfere with my ability to wholeheartedly concur with the new belief system. These techniques included scrupulously adhered-to sessions of meditation and visualization, with the goal being to increase my body's tolerance for the toxic agents, to maximize their destruction of the unwanted cells in the body, and to train my mind and body to expect success in each stage of the event.

These were no small adjustments to make. I was then, as I am now, an unyieldingly logical person. It would have been nearly preferable for me to die, rather than to be duped out of desperation. I knew that the orange liquid in the metal carrying case posed a danger to every cell in my body. The trick was to convince myself that I could instruct my healthy, useful cells to decline to absorb any of that orange juice, while letting those mutant cells bathe and drink to their heart's delight. I drew pictures of the chemotherapy drugs hugging my organs while poisoning leukemia cells. I held conferences with the captain of the heroic orange cavalry, riding his orange horse. We planned elaborate strategies and designed fantastic orange laser weaponry. Our plans were coordinated with the antiterrorist SWAT specialists of my immune system. I called them into action, educated them in the tactics of the enemy, and sent them on bloody missions to destroy the vulnerable foe. I then visualized my immune system cells disposing of the destroyed opponent. I went to sleep each night to the tape-recorded voice of a legendary figure from the healing arts. A woman I'd never met, who told me every night that she loved me, and that everything that was happening to me was for the greatest good. I even had conversations with a mental image of myself twenty years into the future, who guided me, and assured me that he was the proof of my inevitable survival.

This middle-aged manifestation of myself wasn't difficult to conjure up. Just as my spirit was being rejuvenated by leaps and bounds, my physical being was hurtling along in the opposite direction. While I'd open my eyes from every meditation session having regressed a little further into the youthful era of curiosity and discovery, I'd be met by an image in the mirror of a rapidly aging man. Each day I'd become more debilitated, a bit slower, my posture more stooped. My hairline was receding hourly, and the pace of its retreat could be manipulated simply by reaching up and removing a clump of hairs with my fingers. With that simple gesture I'd scroll forward on my lifeline to see myself reflected back from five, ten, twenty years down the road. The mirror became the window through which these different chronological incarnations would greet each other and try each day to build a new bridge to reconnect the ever-widening chasm between.

The techniques I learned were a result of the reading I was doing. Immediately after the diagnosis I had begun collecting what would soon grow into a library of inspirational books and articles. This collection started with a few well-intentioned gifts from friends and relatives, but soon exploded with the addition of obscure pamphlets promoting alternative cures; letters from long-lost friends; letters from the friends of those friends; all giving hazy anecdotal testimonials of miraculous recoveries, typed out on worn typewriters and scrawled over page after page of personal stationery. Several of the submissions contained audiocassettes of speeches given by the New

Age gurus of the day, or bootleg tapes of their smaller support group meetings. These tapes were often referred to as if they were treasured gems of the underground holistic healing circuit. Their owners would pass them on to me with the solemn reverence of a devoted Dead Head, certain that it was *this* tape, of *this* particular performance, that would make me see the light, and change my life forever.

Some of this stuff was brought in at my request — I was aware of and eager to read what Norman Cousins had to say about illness. I devoured his book *Anatomy of an Illness*, and found even more valuable information in his later one *The Healing Heart*. In these books, Cousins explicitly states many of the discoveries I myself was making. Namely, that disease was not the only obstacle to be overcome. The institutions supposedly devoted to making the sick well could easily exhaust the stamina of the heartiest souls. Even before I'd read his books, when I had first arrived on the twelfth floor of the hospital, the first thing I was told was that I couldn't keep the VCR I'd brought with me. Plugging it in was "against the rules," as the only available electrical outlets were reserved for emergency medical equipment, in case its use became necessary. I learned then, and reading about Norman Cousins's experiences confirmed for me, that my ability to survive was going to be closely related to my willingness to disobey. I also started to try to emulate others of Cousins's survival techniques, such as getting the nursing staff to consolidate their repeated requests for my bodily fluids.

As invaluable as I found the Cousins books, there was another small blue paperback whose pages I adopted as my personal manifesto. The book became my Bible. *Getting Well Again*, by Stephanie and O. Carl Simonton, was the book that planted most of these ideas in my head.

Carl Simonton was a radiologist in the Dallas area who became intrigued with the question of why two individuals with nearly identical diagnoses and treatment protocols might come to have completely different treatment histories over the course of their illnesses. Some patients recovered and lived long lives, while others succumbed almost immediately, in spite of identical interventions. Dr. Simonton focused his investigations on the emotional makeup of these individuals; the stresses in their lives prior to diagnosis; and their ability and willingness to reexamine their life choices and belief systems. One of the key theories put forth by Carl and Stephanie Simonton in *Getting Well Again,* and later by Dr. Bernie Siegel in his book *Love, Medicine and Miracles,* is the idea of "taking responsibility for one's illness." Each of their books, as well as many others', speaks at great length about lives lived out of sync with an individual's true desires, and how easily we can come to accept roles for ourselves that are not necessarily of our own choosing. The books recommend adopting an attitude toward illness as one of being presented with an opportunity. The reader is encouraged to view the illness as a message to be heeded, a state of *dis*-ease in the body, and to strive to break free of commitments and responsibilities that are causing feelings of despair and hopelessness. A great deal of space in these books is devoted to what might make up the curriculum for a basic assertiveness-training seminar.

I have no idea what caused me to develop leukemia. My own intuition tells me that growing up three miles from a nuclear power plant is probably not the best way to avoid health problems. Nor would I recommend the game my brother and sister and I used to play every Tuesday evening in the summers. That was the night when, in the humid, glowing, sunset swelter, The Fog Man made his rounds.

The Fog Man wasn't a man at all. Or, while there was a man involved, he wasn't the object of our interest. What captivated us was the small green tractorlike vehicle with the engine that revved like machine-gun fire. Each Tuesday evening, after the sun had set but before darkness fell, the sputtering of the engine would build as The Fog Man approached. His tractor moved slowly along the side of the winding road, while the elevated chute protruding from the right back side of the rumbling machine spewed insecticide in billowing plumes up into the shrubs and trees.

We would wait, listening for The Fog Man's call. When we heard him rounding the bend, his truck whining higher as it struggled to climb the hill, we would sneak out one of the seven back doors of the large house we'd dubbed "Somanydoors." Hiding in the bushes, we would watch as The Fog Man pulled over onto the dirt shoulder of the road and, slowing down for his pass by the homes of the subscribers to his service, blasted the moist, white smoke from the asshole of his engine. We would pull our T-shirts over our mouths and noses, and, giggling and shrieking, we would run and play in the mist. We would follow him down the road, from house to house, trying to get as close to the thickest meat of the fog as we could without actually shoving our faces into the chute itself. We would become lost in the clouds, hearing each other's laughter but unable to locate one another with our eyes, until we escaped, choking on the sweet fumes, spent and out of breath. We would collapse on top of each other, bragging about our bravery, and vowing ever more daring stunts for the next week, when The Fog Man would return.

Seventeen years later, in the midst of my treatments, I celebrated a birthday with a small group of friends who had all grown up within a few miles of each other in the lower Hudson Valley. In the group of six men and women, all under the age of thirty, three of them had been treated for some form of cancer. I myself was aware of two other young people living in the same area who had been or were currently ill. Since none of these cancers were "related" in terms of their location in the body, this shocking outcropping would never be classified as a cancer "cluster," and so, never investigated.

Of course, even if there were a clear, documentable cause for these illnesses, there would still be the question of why these particular people became ill when so many were exposed to the same environmental factors. What Drs. Simonton and Siegel were offering was a sense of power and control. A sense of simple cause and effect. While all the doctors were emphasizing the randomness of my history, and, more important, of my hope for recovery, here was a way of thinking that offered me some influence over the course of events. Even if I wasn't sure, it made a certain amount of sense to me to simply *assign* a cause for the illness. Just pick one that felt emotionally vivid, and work on changing that particular aspect of my life. At the very least, I would be sending to myself the powerful subliminal message that I was working toward gaining the very greatest potential for healing. And, although I could never be positive, there was always the possibility that I might actually hit upon a contributing factor, and by acting upon it, substantially enhance my chances. If the way that I had responded to the stress of the world included cultivating a cancer, then changing the way that I experienced my life should alter the chemistry and make for a less fertile environment. Indeed, according to Simonton's thinking, one's belief systems were simply choices themselves, to be eagerly embraced for as long as they proved beneficial, and then discarded and replaced when they no longer served to enhance the quality of one's life. He saw a change of convictions as nothing more than a change of outfits, or hairstyles. I figured, "Hey, it seems to work for a lot of politicians."

And so began the propaganda campaign. With myself as maestro and Jackie as devoted lieutenant, minions of scouts and messengers were dispatched to find and retrieve any and all accounts of long shot victories. There were no criteria as to the field of reference; these didn't have to be replicas of my own predicament. Of course, nothing would have soothed me more than to have had a visit from someone who had conquered precisely what I was facing, but I was starved enough to appreciate much humbler morsels. Tell me about the "infertile" couple who were celebrating the birth of their first child; read to me about the runner who was told she'd never walk again. The topic didn't even have to be related to health in any way. My life was being transformed by sportscasters who would announce certain defeat for teams losing by margins that had never been surmounted before. Each time I witnessed one of these premature eulogies shattered by an unexpected comeback, I took it as a personal message that my duty was to provide the world with yet another example, this one more miraculous than any that had come before.

A lot of the propaganda handed to me was brought in or sent unsolicited. Some of these items were wondrous accounts of spontaneous healings that had supposedly occurred. Occasionally, these would be described in letters, written by the subjects themselves, who happened to be people that I had known or been introduced to in my life. One woman, an ex-girlfriend of a good friend of mine, wrote me a long letter describing her history of cervical cancer. Soon after her diagnosis, she began a journey of investigation, delving into many different types of spiritual healing and emotional therapies. She told me, in her letter, about coming to terms with the sexual abuse she had suffered as a child, and how, after one particular day of deep contemplation and cleansing tears, a small mass of tissue had dropped out of her body, and no cancer was ever found again. I became fascinated with these accounts. Hearing about them, reading documentation of them, boosted my spirits tremendously. I remained skeptical about a lot of what I was hearing, but there were also stories that were compelling and hard to dispute. In the hours that I spent pondering them, fondling them, I would luxuriate in their reassurance, relishing the inspiration they offered.

This sudden shift in my demeanor and outlook took a lot of people who knew me by surprise. Friends, relatives, anyone who came to visit would enter the room slowly, cautiously. Their body language seemed to suggest both an empathic concern for me and my privacy in such a difficult time as well as a not so easily disguised expression of "Oh, Jesus. Just what am I in for when I enter this room?"

Not that I blame anyone for that. I can think of nothing that I would have dreaded more than having to call on someone just diagnosed with a horrible disease. I'm barely better equipped to handle that kind of thing now. It's not that I don't like sick people. It's not that at all. I just hate to be around them.

My visitors, once the treatment had begun, were met not with grief and agony, but with a transformed individual who would regularly give long, detailed inspirational lectures. I would chastise anyone whose grief showed through for bringing me down, assuring them that I was not only confident I would survive, but that I could now envision a much more fulfilling life for myself as a result of the trauma. I was exhibiting a vigor and a spirituality that had not previously existed in me. I was, in some sense, brought to life for the first time at the prospect of having it taken away.

I had been leading a life of not so quiet discontent for some time, I would explain, and now my life at last had a clear, well-defined purpose. First, to simply survive; and then, to learn to live my life in a manner much truer to my fantasies of what I wanted life to be. Not that there wasn't plenty of despair still surfacing, but I was also experiencing a euphoric high from the anticipation of how amazing my existence could be if I could reclaim it after having endured the agony of its apparent loss. I spent hours fantasizing about how it would be, if I ever got well, to run into some of the people from my old life again. I swore that I would pour my heart out to them, to let them know what I had learned. That life on the planet Earth was the sweetest candy, the milkiest pearl. That to have a day to spend with someone you love and to expect another one tomorrow had become the most beautiful, lush, and soothing privilege to me. I think that not a few friends left the hospital during this time relieved to have been spared a more mournful scene; inspired to reapproach their own lives and opportunities; and just a little concerned for my mental stability and my connection to reality.

I even went so far as to employ the services of several psychics.

Laurel Starr was a psychic healer living in Tribeca, whom my friend Didi told me about. I scheduled Laurel to come to the hospital for a first session. When the day arrived, I had a pretty clear picture of a rounded, middle-aged, gypsy-looking woman that I'd spot as soon as I saw her. The door to my room swung open and Laurel looked at my girlfriend in the chair and said, "Jackie?"

Wow. Pretty fucking psychic, I thought. Jackie said, "Laurel? Laurel Kummermann?"

It turned out they had gone to grade school together. Laurel Kummermann had turned into Laurel Starr, and, according to Jackie, her nose had been revamped as much as her name. Well, however she had done it, she was gorgeous. A blond psychic bombshell.

Laurel and I began having regular sessions together. She became my spiritual guide, in a way. The sessions were like therapy, like a shrink, but with the emphasis on intuitions, mine and hers, with a hands-on healing included with each one. Anyone who saw Laurel was astonished by her beauty, which was accentuated by the provocative way she dressed for her visits to the hospital. She'd often arrive with several bags from Bloomingdale's in tow. Lots of jokes were made about what went on during our sessions, how come I seemed so content afterward, and how come I needed to go to sleep right after each one.

The reality was that amazing things were accomplished when we saw each other. Laurel saw aspects of me that I had not been aware of, and related them to the disease I was fighting. Laurel spoke to me about her impressions of a soul that was clinging to childhood, refusing to mature. She described me as an individual who needed to discover that he was capable of surviving his own mistakes, and to then go on and learn to relish them. Laurel was able to predict serious medical episodes, as did the dreams that I would relate to her. She also told me a great deal about her personal life, which included a husband and a Sicilian boyfriend, both of whom lived with her — together. I started to fantasize about Laurel. A lot.

This brought up some problems. First of all, I was really sick by this time. I was heavily drugged and depending on blood transfusions to keep me alive. If my counts were down and a transfusion was due, just walking across the room could make my heart pound so hard that I imagined the nurses in the hallway could hear it. In the hours after a fresh infusion of blood cells had perked me up, I would get incredibly turned on from thinking about my guru, Laurel; even more, my body seemed to sense that it was being poisoned by the chemotherapy, and this produced a level of horniness that I'd never felt before. My theory was that the body sensed its own destruction and had one priority: *REPRODUCE.*

And then there was the problem of Laurel's "psychic powers." She had often spoken of her own trouble of having her thoughts confused by messages she would get as other people thought about her; or of how difficult it was for her to go out in public because her mind would be assaulted by other people's thoughts leaking into her head. I began to have uncontrollable sexual fantasies about her whenever she was around, always accompanied by the horror that she knew exactly what I was thinking all the time.

A few times, I braved my fear and actually masturbated in my hospital room — in spite of the fact that I was afraid my heart might literally explode, or that I'd have a stroke if I were to have an orgasm. That, and the fact that I was thinking about my psychic at the time, a guilt that I guess was equal to fantasizing about a priest or a nun — except that my psychic might actually be assaulted by images of me jerking off in my hospital room, inches from death, while she was making breakfast at home with her husband and her Sicilian boyfriend. I started hoping that he wasn't psychic as well.

I still find that whole phase of my life terribly difficult to describe or to reconcile with who I was before or who I have been since. The truth is, I can't muster the kind of optimistic attitude I had then while trying to pick out a good cantaloupe today. That's why I regarded my newfound optimism as a form of opportunism. I was able to incorporate, to absorb a system of thinking completely laugh-able to me. I was able to exploit some odd mechanism in my brain that allowed me to reprogram it for the purposes of maximizing my survival potential. I think that I knowingly brainwashed myself. And I think that the part of me that was brainwashed knowingly allowed it to happen. That kind of duplicity was, for me, absolutely essential.

If my friends were perplexed by my soaring spirit, the hospital staff was downright bewildered. And most of them seemed determined to bring me right back down to Earth.

I would begin each day by pushing aside the chairs to create some open space in the cramped half a hospital room. Semiprivate, in hospital double-speak. As if privacy isn't something whose very nature is either absolute or nonexistent. Then I'd put on earphones with a fifteen-foot-long cord. I'd roll the IV pole that I was attached to, along with all the bottles dangling from it, across the hospital room and I would dance.

I had brought a collection of my favorite, most inspirational music to the hospital and I would close the door to my room, close my eyes, and dance and forget where I was. I'd get caught up in the power of the music and let it surge through me. I would try to imagine that the energy being released in each drum beat, in every bass note, was being passed on to me and being stored up as part of my life force. I'd begin to break a sweat as I would let my body swing and gyrate more and more, giving myself over to the rhythms. I'd look up and be startled to see the door to the room open. Two or three nurses would be standing there, huddled together and staring at me, with looks of concern and confusion on their faces. When they saw that I had discovered them there, they would snicker and whisper to each other as they walked away.

That was on a good day. More than once I was torn from my blissful trance by the scolding voice of a nurse who hissed, "What are you doing?"

"Dancing," I'd say, surprised that it wasn't obvious.

Then, with a tone and manner of someone doing a campy Nurse Ratched impersonation, she'd charge into the room saying, "Well, I've got to make up the bed. You should be eating your breakfast."

For those very reasons I started hanging a sign on my door requesting that I not be disturbed at certain times of the day. I may have been paranoid. But I suspected that if dancing was a threatening activity to them, they might not understand seeing my psychic healer waving her hands over my body. Or my hypnotherapist drumming in his subliminal messages. Or my psychiatrist taking notes calmly while I sobbed in a chair.

A huge part of my daily life in the hospital became covert and had to be hidden. Even little rituals. Laurel Starr had instructed Jackie on how to "charge" my food before each meal. First, Jackie would go out and get some take-out food from the neighborhood. I very rarely ate the hospital food, ever since my first day there, when I was served Kellogg's cereal, replete with BHA and BHT to "insure freshness." Jackie would close her eyes and meditate. She'd concentrate on forming a healing, purifying white light in her mind. Then she'd send this heat and energy into her hands, hold her hands over my food, and shoot all those hot, happening rays out and into my meal.

I loved this. I mean I *really* loved this, and I really got into it. This was something that I could sink my teeth into, both literally and figuratively. I was having a hard time eating to begin with, due to the nausea from the chemotherapy, and this gave me a reason to make myself eat, as well as a fantastic visceral image of strength and empowerment with every mouthful. For hours after each meal, I'd feel the warmth of Jackie's love and her healing prayers being carried through my bloodstream to all my hungry cells.

Sometimes, the gifts Jackie and I were given were not terribly well thought out. Luckily for me, Jackie was in a position where she could exist financially without full-time work. She had not only become my constant companion and guardian, but also, after working twelve-hour shifts by my side in the hospital, Jackie would stay up much of the night screening the books and tapes being brought by friends. She was regularly passing on the materials that she thought would lift my spirits, while sifting out those stories whose messages weren't consistent with the mind-set we were trying to create. There was rarely any discussion of those books; they would simply disappear with Jackie for her nightly reading, never to return, and never to be inquired about. The balance between the deception we were attempting to create for ourselves and our awareness of that deception was a delicate one. The denial of all doubt-provoking stimuli was a job that required enormous attention and vigilance.

Occasionally, our defense would be caught off guard, or overwhelmed. I was once given by a close friend a book called *We the Victors*, which I'd heard about and was eager to read. It was described as an intense account of several individuals who had survived devastating cancers, and it was supposed to be an inspirational, life-affirming, remarkable testament to the human spirit. After leaving the hospital late the night before, Jackie came back the next morning looking nervous and shaken. While it was obvious that something was wrong, she wouldn't tell me what it was. I asked her if she had the book for me, to which she curtly replied, "No." Day after day, I continued to ask Jackie about the book. Her answer expanded, somewhat, into "You don't want to read it."

It was weeks before I could get Jackie to tell me what she'd read. Apparently, interspersed with stories of amazing recoveries, of hardships overcome, there was one tragic account. As Jackie told me the story of a nurse who had fallen in love with a young leukemia patient, only to watch him die an extremely frightening and painful death, she started to cry.

"It was awful," she said. Her voice was startlingly high-pitched, the words barely audible amidst the crying that had taken control of her breathing. "It was really bad." It was the first time that Jackie had shown any weakness to me since the diagnosis, and I suddenly realized how ridiculous I had been to think that anyone could maintain her level of composure amidst everything she was dealing with. I had never seen Jackie as upset as she was, and it terrified me. I had come to depend on her totally to shield me from all those forces that could be controlled, all the more since there seemed to be so many over which we had none. If Jackie's strength were to falter, I wondered, who would be there to take her place?

Beneath the fear, I was overwhelmed by sadness. I could see on Jackie's face what I recognized as disappointment. I watched her turn, in one moment, from my hero, who had convinced me that she (and therefore I) was invincible, into a frightened child who was ashamed of her failure to subdue her own terror. I was able to recognize, as a result of my own disappointment over what I saw as my family's lack of awareness, that just as I needed someone whom I could trust to catch me if I were to collapse, Jackie would also at times need to abandon her stance of strength and reveal the helplessness that she was feeling herself. I held her as she cried and, with not a clue as to how I would deliver the goods, I promised her everything was going to be all right.

When communication between my parents and me had become almost nonexistent, when any attempt at conversation bulged with a tension on the verge of bursting, I got a card in the mail from my father. The card was one of a series of Japanese-style black-and-white line drawings my father had made years before. Many of the paintings in the series are hauntingly evocative, using the fewest lines possible to impart reams of emotional information about the subjects. This illustration showed three faceless figures, obviously a parent and two children, due to the size of the figures and the pose. The taller figure was in the center, while the two smaller figures, each with an arm draped protectively around their shoulders, were being hugged in toward the looming presence of the larger body. Not only hadn't I received a letter from my father in years, but I hadn't seen his handwriting in nearly as long. When I opened the card and read what my father had written to me, before I had even absorbed one word of his message, I was thrown back in time to my childhood, sitting at his desk, reading his emphatic notes. The urgency of the words back then was so apparent, even though their meaning was lost on me. This letter, though, I understood.

My Dear Son,

Although it shouldn't wait until times like these to clarify our feelings for each other and of the lives we lead, this has happened to me and I assume to you as well.

The depth of my love for you astounded me. So instead of just hitting a new low in pain this past month I also hit a new high in awareness. Not only of myself but of you and your life.

I see you now as a man with extraordinary inner strength, with the capacity to look into yourself and bring to an extreme situation all that the mind and heart can muster. More than that, you brought all of us up by your words and actions when you were most down.

I admire you more than any person I have ever known.

Thank you for being my son.

Dad.

I cried when I read it. I still have it, and I cry every time I read it now.

*   *   *

As I continued to get sicker and sicker, with one infection after another, the hospital clergy started bidding for my soul. On every doorway to every room there was a nameplate to identify who was inside. These nameplates also indicated whether each patient wanted a newspaper delivered to their room, if so, which newspaper, and included a letter to indicate what their religion was. C,P,J,M. That kind of thing. I guess they got tipped off by the doctors, because whenever my condition deteriorated, I started getting visits from the rabbis.

The rabbis would bring Welch's grape juice, instead of wine, and they'd ask permission to say some prayers with me. They would try to get me to come downstairs to the services in the chapel, and I'd balk and make excuses, all the while thinking that they must also somehow know about my lust for my psychic — as if there was some kind of spiritual information-exchange program, a conspiracy, and they were trying to lure me away from her.

They did propose one thing, however, that I thought was so sweet and innocent that I agreed right away. In the Jewish religion there is something known as the Book of Life. Every birth is recorded in this book, and every event of that life is preordained. Also in the book are the date, the time, and the manner of that person's death. When the time comes, the angel of death is sent, and the soul is escorted to . . . wherever Jewish souls go with the angel of death. In cases of serious illness or injury, a ceremony is sometimes performed as part of the weekend synagogue service. The individual's life is discussed, and a new name is assigned. A birth certificate is filled out, using the date from the Hebrew calendar, and *presto·* with a new name, the person is safe. Unidentifiable. The angel of death goes looking, but he is fooled. Fooled by the cunning of a rabbi from Great Neck.

So I became Chaim. A small price to pay, I thought. But I wondered how many times you could pull that trick before the angel of death caught on. Or, was there more than one angel of death, and were some of them harder to fool than others?

On October 16, 1985, I came walking down the hallway of Sloan-Kettering's twelfth floor. I had gone down to the coffee shop with my sister and Jackie, to try to eat a cheeseburger, French fries, and a chocolate milkshake to make up some of the eleven pounds I had already lost. I'd never weighed more than one-hundred-thirty-three pounds in my life to begin with. Down to one-twenty-two, I was sporting a decidedly scarecrowlike appearance. I was met in the hallway by Debbie Brown, a short, roundish nurse who had been as consistently friendly and encouraging as others had been abusive. Debbie had a huge smile on her face, and she was bouncing up and down like a ten-year-old girl with a secret.

"The doctors are looking for you," she said. "They're in your room."

Earlier that day some bone marrow had been "aspirated," or sucked out, from the back of my hipbone to be examined and checked for any leukemia. If the marrow was clean, then the first, or the "induction," course of chemotherapy (as in "inducing" remission) would be considered successful. Then I could go home and take a month off before moving on to rounds two and three, known as "consolidation chemo."

This bone marrow aspirate and bone biopsy was a procedure that I had first experienced on the day of diagnosis with Dr. Nixon. In the five weeks since, it had already gone a long way toward becoming what it would remain for the next few years: something like the overgrown six-foot psychotic bully from third grade who decides one day, out of the blue, that you're his best friend and can never be out of his sight. You walk around everywhere in the shadow of this hulking beast, always fearful but never knowing exactly when he's going to snap and punch you in the face.

The procedure is done most often by a doctor working alone, or with a nurse assisting. A table is laid ready with a set of several slides, and a package, sealed for sterility, is snapped open. Inside are the tools, the instruments, that the doctor will use. While you lie on your stomach, with your pants pulled halfway down the length of your backside and your head turned to one side, the doctor presses firmly on either side of the base of your spine to find an easily accessible bone outcropping. If you reach back and feel the bones that stick out on either side of the spine, right below your pant waist, you'll find the spot they're looking for. The doctor then injects into the skin, with a hypodermic needle, an anesthetic called lidocaine. This produces an intense, but short-lived, stinging sensation, after which the doctor pushes the needle in deeper and deeper, injecting more lidocaine and causing more stinging, until the needle is pressing against the bone. The needle is then removed and set aside, and, while the doctor vigorously rubs the flesh under the injection site to hasten the effects of the anesthetic, he will attempt to engage you in conversation.

Now is the time, you see, when all the warm patter, the compassionate human contact, that has been so craved but absent from the brusque daily visits to the bedside is offered. Now, with the doctor behind you and out of sight. Now, with your face smashed into a pillow, and your naked ass sticking up in the air. And without fail I accepted, gratefully, every time.

With the appetizer finished, the main course consists of a long, thick needle being *screwed,* first through your skin, and then into the back of your hipbone, with the doctor, often a two-hundred-pound man, *pressing* down on you with all his strength. This isn't so much terribly painful as terrifying. I was never able to stop myself from imagining the needle somehow snapping off inside me, or, worse still, suddenly meeting a soft spot and smashing all the way through me until it ripped out the front side.

But those things never happened. When the needle was in deep enough, the doctor would screw on a large syringe, and pull back, to suck some of the marrow out from inside my bones. *That* was painful. No anesthetic had reached inside my bones, and, since there is a pressure vacuum inside these bones of ours, the deep, dull pain would reach down, down, down the leg, into the foot, into the insides of the very inside of the self. Yes, into the very marrow of one's bones, as the saying goes, the doctor would go drilling, tunneling to find a lode more precious than any gem deep inside the Earth. If you can imagine what it might feel like to a bowl of chocolate pudding if you sucked some of it up through a straw, that's what it feels like to have a bone marrow aspirate.

For dessert, the bone biopsy. Many doctors also find it a useful diagnostic tool to break off a tiny piece of bone to examine under the microscope. For this, another tool is screwed into the needle already in your body, and, once it's in place, the doctor *shakes* the whole gizmo, with your body attached to it, quite vigorously. I have discovered, through my experiences with leukemia, that I have got very, very tough bones. I've had them complimented by several doctors in several different states. I've been told how lucky I am to have such strong bones, how tough it would be to break such strong bones, as I've been tossed and thrown around like a doll impaled on a spear.

When I walked into the room I saw, in separate corners, Dr. Zweig and my parents. Everyone in the room was standing. My marrow had been drawn several hours earlier, and we had all been waiting, like a death row prisoner and his kin, to hear whether I was to be granted a stay of execution or not. If the results showed that remission had not been successfully induced, there would be no choice but to begin the month-long process over immediately and try again. Either that or go home to die. I tried my best to mask my awareness of what I was asking, as I faced Dr. Zweig and said, "Good news?"

"Yeah. Pretty good," he barely squeaked.

"What do you mean 'Pretty good'? Is it in remission or what?"

"Yeah, yeah." He seemed to be answering begrudgingly, using as little breath as was required to make a sound that might be accepted as a reply. "I'd say we have a very young, new remission marrow. Don't get your hopes up too high, though. Still a *loong* way to go."

Then he added, "You know, that was one of the easiest inductions I've ever seen here."

I couldn't tell if he was congratulating me on a job well done, or telling me "You just wait. We're gonna get you next time around."

At the time when I wound up in the hospital, I wouldn't have considered myself to be the most widely loved or lovable actor on the planet. My way of dealing with the frustrations of the business, the inevitable envy and resentments of watching others transcend my own success, had become the habit of telling anyone who would listen that I was *the* single-most brilliant actor alive in New York City. It was just that I had to have *someone* speaking about me in those terms, even if I was the only one that I could get to do it.

In spite of this, visitors flooded in to see me. The blood bank of the hospital was deluged with people clamoring to have their fluids drawn, stored, and transfused. My mother and her sister had formed a fund to take donations to be used to pay medical and living expenses for me and the family. Several people in the theater community banded together and organized benefit performances of two shows running off-Broadway that raised a great deal of money and drew a wide assortment of people, many of whom didn't even know me. They all wanted to know how they could help, and I'm sure they were surprised when their offers were accepted, and they were told that Jackie and I had just bought ten gallons of "hint of peach," and the apartment walls were waiting. While I lay in the hospital, a group of my friends, both close and merely distant, painted my home for my release and arrival. Each day Jackie would tell me who had shown up, and I would be so moved that I could barely breathe.

I don't know how to describe it except to say that the ending of the movie *It's a Wonderful Life* had suddenly jumped out of the TV set and become my reality. Clarence the angel's inscription to George

Bailey that "no man is a failure who has friends" was etched into my soul and comforted me in my anguish over having been torn from my competitive race against so many perceived opponents. Opponents who were now rushing to be by my side, to shop for my girlfriend, to wash our clothes, or just hold our hands. I still see my life, the fact that I'm alive, as a kind of crazy community project. I like to be around so that the people who helped out can see their work. Their blood runs in my veins. Literally. I have my life because other people pumped some of theirs into me.

And this relatively easy, love-filled ride that I got my first time through really seemed to piss off the people who had led me to expect worse. It was like the doctors were angry at me for proving them wrong by doing better than they'd predicted. As my family and I celebrated the first success in the quest to win back my life, Dr. Zweig was in the corner pouting. He looked like a crusty old war vet who can't stand to see some snot-nosed, cherry private escape the front lines without watching at least one of his buddies get his head blown off.

There seems to be a great fear of something known as "false hope." I've heard the phrase used by doctors and nurses again and again, in very self-congratulatory ways, as if, by exterminating it, they were providing a great philanthropic service to the community.

Now, I scratch my way through this world as nothing if not a pessimist, and I will state, unequivocally, that there is no such thing as false hope. It's an oxymoron. It can't exist.

Hope has no connotations of certainty. Hope carries no assurance of success. Hope is the one thing in this world that can never, ever, be false. Hope is just exactly what it says. A longing. A desire. Is there such a thing as a false, aching desire?

I think, too often, that some doctors are protecting *themselves* from the aching desires, the hope, of their patients. It must be very painful to fail to save the life of someone who never concealed his passion to survive. His hope. Much more painful than the death of a patient willing to hide the intensity of his wish. If only they could learn what a potent source of energy they're wasting.

After Zweig had left the room, after my family and I had finished with our hugs and our tears, I walked back out to the hospital corridor. I saw families clustered outside the rooms weeping. I took a number of hard looks at the fear in the faces of the husbands and wives, sons and daughters, nieces, grandchildren, nephews. Never was the terror more pungent, the anxiety more palpable, than when they were searching for hope in the face of a doctor.

I walked down the hallway past the nurses' station. I remembered that the purpose of a hospital is simply to provide around-the-clock nursing care for a great number of people at once. Doctors are secondary to the equation. They wield most of the power but do very little of the hands-on care. Some of the nurses that I saw through the glass, and many of the nurse's aides, had proven to be genuine exceptions to the hard rule of most of the higher-ups. Olivia Squire and Gisella Sanchez-Ortiz, Debbie Brown and Sharon — several others whose names I never learned — had all lived up to the classical images of generous, compassionate, and devoted nurses. There was also Dr. Pisters, a Canadian woman who, at twenty-three, was younger than I was. We sat up together many nights, sharing stories of being the youngest person in our separate professional peer groups. We had laughed together, as she haltingly applied her medical knowledge and struggled through procedures with me. I had endured most of them dozens of times while I was her first attempt at their application. I had no problem with her admitted lack of expertise and appreciated her allowing me to instruct her on how to best approach them from a patient's point of view. She, much to her credit, had freely encouraged me in my daily battles, often offering me favorable comparisons between my condition and others she had seen come and go. When Dr. Pisters heard of my remission, she jumped up and waved to me through the glass window of the nurses' station. She shrieked and burst into tears of joy. Two older doctors, attending physicians, on either side of her, immediately shot her ferociously scolding stares, and she looked away from me, wiped her eyes, and went back to work at the computer.

As I walked the hall, swearing that October 16 would forever be my new birthday, it seemed clear to me that those who were closest to the patients for the greatest amount of time were the most helpful and caring. I know that I got the most encouragement from the men and women who filled my water pitcher and emptied the urine container that hung on my bed. My personal hydrationists. All day and through the deep night they would visit me. Always with sympathy, compassion, and tales of those who had triumphed. Many times, from many mouths, in several different lilting accents, I heard the same mission spoken: "It's my job, mon, to go see de patient after de doctor get tru wit him. Dat way I tell de patient he don have to die like de doctor tell him he do."

FAMILY AFFAIRS

As a nonpracticing Jewish man, I was, at first, bewildered by a vision I had of myself, crucified on a hospital bed, sacrificing my life for the sins of my family. If I was going to have a religious epiphany, couldn't I at least stay within the faith? I had, though, in recent days, been feeling more and more troubled by underexamined memories from my childhood. Periods from my growing up that had never been discussed, and events that had been treated as if they had never occurred.

I first met Dr. Yehuda Nir, a psychiatrist, only a week or two after being diagnosed with leukemia. His name came to me from Jackie, who had gotten it from her brother, who had gotten it from his friend, who happened to be a psychotherapist. This was how things got done.

Our first meeting took place in his office on Park Avenue. I had never visited a psychiatrist before, but even in my ignorance I was surprised by the small, drab, gray-green waiting room whose window looked out only onto an air shaft that was grayer still.

Dr. Nir was a small man, either of a nondescript physical nature or simply not vivid enough for me to form a clear impression upon a first meeting. He was balding and dressed crisply in trousers, shirt, and tie, and he spoke with what, at the time, sounded to me like a parody of a psychiatrist's mysterious European accent. Nir had once been on staff at Sloan-Kettering himself, but he now worked out of his own office, where he treated what seemed to be a steady stream of Hasidic Jews and wrote self-help books with his wife. Our first meeting consisted mostly of gentle questioning by Dr. Nir, as he prodded me for information about my idols while growing up and asked for brief descriptions of my childhood and the happenings of the past few weeks. The intensity of the sessions picked up quickly though, as he began to probe my beliefs about myself and the world around me.

Nir began to stress that my perception of things was not necessarily in complete agreement with an absolute reality. He would correct me when I despondently referred to the "miracle" I would need to ever see my fortieth birthday. "Lots of people get well," he said. "And they stay well." I had no idea if this was true or not. But it made me feel a lot better to hear him say it.

Then Dr. Nir would remind me of the ways that I had been taught, throughout my life, to scrupulously avoid danger. To always consider and prepare for misfortune, for catastrophe. I was, in fact, so entrenched in my accepted way of thinking that I would argue with him over the significance of bizarre Handler family rituals.

For example, it was an unquestioned practice that whenever both of my parents went away together on a plane, they would leave a sealed envelope for their children, "in case the plane goes down." This envelope was said to contain the information that we would need in the event of their deaths, such as the location of safe-deposit boxes and wills, the names and numbers of lawyers, and, we were told, the envelope was to be opened only in the event that both of them were killed.

All of my life, this had seemed perfectly logical to me. Not until I started to question, with the help of my therapist, the messages behind this drama did I even consider any alternative methods of action. Such as, instead of turning every parental plane trip into a potential tragedy — with the envelope serving as a constant reminder, from departure to return, that we might never see each other again — simply leaving a permanent file in a drawer somewhere with all the information necessary in case of emergency. It was only during my therapy with Dr. Nir that I finally decided that this preoccupation with disaster was somehow desired by my parents because, in spite of my asking them to refrain from leaving the "farewell note" in the future, upon their next vacation, there was the envelope once again, sitting prominently on the kitchen table.

"I'm going to open it and see what it says," I told my sister and brother.

"I don't think they want you to do that," Lowell said.

It was astonishing to witness grown, adult children unflinchingly obeying destructive commands. I, myself, was frightened to assert my independence and blatantly disregard my parents' wishes, even though they had disregarded mine by, once again, leaving the ghostly reminder of their mortality to stand in for them in their absence. When I opened the envelope my anger dissolved. It melted, instead, into a lukewarm puddle of sadness. Inside was a sweet-natured, upbeat good-bye message, written in my mother's hand, wishing us wonderful lives amid her directions of how to arrange all of her and my father's affairs.

How many times, since my childhood, has she done this? I wondered. And at what cost to herself? Why would a parent want to sit down and deliberately imagine a scenario in which they must say good-bye to their children, over and over during their lifetime? And to impose the ghoulish fantasy on the offspring as well? But this was the first time that any of these questions had occurred to me, and for the first time I was thinking that I would have to learn how to protect myself from that kind of chronic preoccupation with the worst that might be in store. I would have to closely examine and adjust my own ingrained reactions to living, and to the risks involved in it. I would also have to guard myself against the constant pressure within the family to continue to uphold the structure that had been in place since before my birth.

I had no idea how difficult this process would prove to be. I was working so furiously myself, desperate to distance myself from whatever traits might have made me "susceptible" to the illness, that anyone would have had a hard time keeping up. I was, by the time I checked back into the hospital for round three, actively working with both Dr. Nir and Laurel Starr, usually twice a week each. I was also seeing another psychiatrist, Dr. John Patten, whom I dubbed the "death therapist" due to his specialty of helping patients and families deal with issues surrounding life-threatening illness. My parents were eager enough to preserve some family unity that they agreed to meet regularly as a group to try to discuss the anger tearing us apart. While I was enraged at them for the awkwardness of some of their early attempts to assist me, they were angry at me for turning on them when they were trying their best to help. I was seeing Dr. Patten once a week with my family, as well as having an occasional private visit to help me master the technique of self-hypnosis.

In addition to my hypnotherapy, my "death therapy," my family therapy, my personal therapy, and my psychic, I was usually consulting simultaneously with any number of nutritionists, astrologists, massage and aroma therapists, as well as working on my own to come up with any insights that might, if not lead to an actual advantage, give me the perception of having one in my fight.

From my earliest awareness, I had felt a compulsion to bring pleasure to the adults around me. My brother's Tourette syndrome had, quite typically, first manifested itself as severe behavioral problems. Hyperactivity, obsessive-compulsive behavior, all kinds of perplexing, frustrating symptoms with no apparent explanation other than some form of psychological disturbance. He had, from an extremely young age, been carted to psychiatrists, and even, occasionally, been prescribed medications to "calm him down." This is a terribly common story for people with Tourette. In even the most well-informed and caring families, which ours was, it often takes years to find a doctor knowledgeable enough about the disorder to correctly identify it. This is a dual tragedy in that, not only is the child misunderstood, but the parents, working furiously to give enlightened help, are often unwittingly compounding the problems by trying to convince a neurologically impaired child, under orders of a physician, that they are emotionally ill.

Being the youngest of three, for most of my childhood I witnessed an older, tormented child venting his rage by tormenting his siblings and his parents. The more my parents tried to control him, or tranquilize him, much to his credit, the harder he would fight back. We took one vacation to Canada that was an absolute nightmare. My parents were quiveringly tense the entire trip, as they tried to get my brother to take the medication that had been prescribed by the latest professional on the case. Lowell had replaced the prescription label on the plastic pharmacy container with a hand-lettered one of his own that read "SICK PILLS," and he insisted that it was not him, but the two barely contained furies in the front seat of the car, who needed tranquilizing.

Since my sister's way of dealing with her confusion growing up was to withdraw from the family, to reject the values and lifestyle that my parents worked endlessly to support, I was aware of a vivid level of pain and difficulty within my parents surrounding my two older siblings. I took it upon myself, with a lot of encouragement from Mom and Dad, to be the bundle of joy. The child whose success came easily and would multiply to the point where the entire family could rest secure. I labored tirelessly to be the one who needed nothing in return; a child who was self-sufficient emotionally and who would provide, at no cost to himself, a ceaseless supply of pleasure and fulfillment to the adults who had been denied it elsewhere. I was to be the "savior" of the family, it was silently agreed. And not only did I keep my needs and fears and vulnerability to myself, but eventually, I stopped being aware that they existed at all.

Years later, as I pondered and probed, as I meditated and spun myself through hypnotic reveries, besides falling deeply in love with life and yearning to recapture my chance at it, I was becoming angry about the ways that I had agreed to live it so far. I thought back and remembered the level of tension in the house when I was in my teens. I remembered a brief span of time at the height of my sister's teenage rebelliousness. My father, never a heavy drinker, had begun to consume more alcohol than before, and he would become frightening in his antagonism toward Lillian. I recalled one episode when, alone in the house with them, I watched him taunt her, threatening her with physical punishment, until she locked herself, crying, into the bathroom. I stood and watched, feeling furious yet helpless, unsure of what I was supposed to do to my father in order to protect my sister from him.

That memory, in turn, reminded me of when my brother had reduced my mother to hysterical tears by refusing, or being unable, to respond to her for hours except to say, over and over, in a high-pitched, teasing voice, "Cheese and crackers . . . cheese and crackers." Lowell had to be seventeen or eighteen years old at the time. Whatever she said to him, whatever he was asked to do, "Cheese and crackers . . . cheese and crackers. Cheese and crackers . . . cheese and crackers." It's not hard to imagine why in medieval times people with Tourette syndrome were thought to be possessed by evil spirits.

I stood outside the kitchen window that day and watched my mother first shriek back at him, in a voice much more Satanic and terrifying than the one he was using, "CHEESE AND CRACKERS!

CHEESE AND CRACKERS!" She then collapsed at the table, sobbing, completely lost as to how to deal with her son. I was never able to forgive myself for not being able to rescue her then, but I couldn't get myself to tell him to stop. It somehow felt as if that would have been too open an admission of the situation, an adult unable to cope with a child, and so being saved by a younger one. Or maybe it was just too ridiculously insane to admit I'd even seen it.

These somewhat traumatic memories, to which I hadn't given much thought for many years, began to occupy more and more of my consciousness. As I attempted to clarify them with some of the newfound insights being gained during my therapy sessions, I felt that I would need the help of some of the other players in order to fully disarm those memories of their potency. And there were other, even darker, secrets I was wrestling with. Amidst my own tentative, fearful attempts at forming sexual relationships, my brother, nearly five years older and much more experienced, had regularly seduced and slept with a succession of my older female friends and girlfriends. Eventually, I confronted him and threatened him with losing his brother forever if he didn't learn to treat me with respect. But much worse were the injuries from a time when I had no way to defend myself. Years earlier, somewhere around the age of eight, when Lowell would have been about twelve or thirteen, I was regularly offered, and given, money for performing sexual acts on my older brother. None of those events had ever been mentioned since.

Though this is, I suppose, a shocking (yet nowadays somewhat excessively revealed) history, I don't recall any feelings of horror or shame from that time. Those responses all came years later, when it seemed terribly out of context to dredge up the perverse experimentations of a younger age. Not only do I believe that what went on is a more common occurrence than is readily admitted, but I'm also not convinced it is an entirely unnatural one — in terms of realizing its potential to occur and in warning children about it and taking steps to protect them from it. We are still, in childhood and as teenagers, before the socialization expected in adulthood is complete, instinctual animals. The attempt to exploit weaker animals by older, stronger ones is something that should be anticipated. The damage is often worsened, in my opinion, by a lack of acknowledgment of the injury. Wounds that might have been superficial are compounded when there is no open discourse about these events and the pain they can cause later, when newfound maturity and comprehension reveal the implications that a child would be unable to perceive. My perception at that young age was that it would have been greedy for me to complain about anything. After all, I was the child with no problems. Attention was needed so much more urgently elsewhere.

I honestly have no idea if any of the emotional traumas of my youth contributed to my developing leukemia. Those events, though troubling, were aberrations on a long, steady graph of tender up-bringing. They have all since been thoroughly discussed and, if not resolved, at least accepted. Put back into the context of my entire upbringing, and considering the families that many others suffer, I was blessed with a charmed childhood, filled with love and genuine expressions of that love. Just as clear, even at the time of my illness, were memories of boundless generosity, as exemplified by gifts of elaborate drum sets and the steady, encouraging presence of my parents at what must have been excruciatingly tedious Little League baseball games. What became tremendously important, though, in my fight to recover from the disease, was that the painful memories of those more haunting, unresolved events *now* felt like burdens to me. When I "woke up" that day, having imagined myself nailed to a hospital bed, wearing a crown of hypodermic needles, I was con-vinced that the effort of maintaining the silence about difficult times in our family history was draining energies that I could not afford to spare. Keeping up the status quo, which had always seemed to be the path of least resistance, now revealed itself to require an enormous amount of exertion. Although I was convinced, at the time, that the role I'd played in the family *had* contributed to a level of exhaustion that left me vulnerable, I was also mindful that more important than discovering the unknowable cause of my illness was the gesture of resigning my post as the keeper of our family secrets. If nothing else, I would once again be demonstrating, to myself, that I was willing to confront any demons, to pursue any path, to give myself the greatest potential for survival.

I sat in sweat pants in the easy chair I'd inherited from my grandparents with the rest of my family gathered around me. My parents had taken me home from the hospital in their car, my brother had driven in from his home north of Manhattan, and my sister had driven in from Pennsylvania. This congregating from various sections of the northeastern United States had become fairly common, as a result of our weekly, or bimonthly, family therapy sessions with John Patten. However, due to the inflammatory issues I intended to broach, I thought the rest of the family might feel less assaulted, less exposed, without any outsiders present. If all went well, I thought, then perhaps the dialogue might be moved into the more structured arena of our therapy sessions together.

The fear that I felt over asking my family to join me in examining our past was as severe as any I had experienced in my life. It was a fear that was different from, yet equal to, the fear I had of losing my life altogether. I have been told many times, by many people, that I am a brave man. The merest mention of the suffering I endured in the treatment of the illness invariably results in proclamations of my bravery from whoever happens to be listening. I expect that anyone who has lain in a hospital bed will recognize what I found to be the most common reaction among visitors when first witnessing the horror of the patient's existence. In hushed and reverential whispers, with tears in their eyes, the visitors shake their heads and say, "Oh, you are such a brave man." And I believe that anyone who has given it much thought would respond in the same way that

I always did: "Running into a burning building when you don't have to, in order to save someone else, is brave. Jumping out a window when you know you'll die if you don't — that's just trying to stay alive." I don't see anything courageous about behavior in situations where there is no choice. But there has been nothing in my life that took more courage than when I gathered my family to ask them to release me from the ties that bound me into remaining the kind of son and brother that they had all come to expect me to be.

The puzzled stares that met my opening declaration of "I'm not what you all think I am, and I'm not what I once believed myself to be," were soon replaced by grimaces and expressions of wounded horror. As I listed very deliberately, one by one, the episodes from my youth that had left painful impressions on me, I tried to carefully make clear my reasons for bringing them up that day. I tried to impress upon everyone that the image of Evan growing up beyond the reach of the pain permeating the rest of the family was the result of a performance that even I hadn't been aware of and that I could no longer continue to pretend. I tried to make it understood that I had endured those events silently as they occurred, but that it had become important to me to be able to speak out loud the fact that I had been hurt by them, even though I hadn't said so at the time. I asked my mother and father, my brother and sister, to please accept responsibility for their own mistakes, their own sins, and I asked them to please, please save me from the guilt I felt over dredging up memories I knew they'd all rather forget. By the time I finished, the huffing and puffing and sighing and shifting coming from my father's side of the room made it clear that he had heard just about enough.

This didn't surprise me. In fact, it had been my worst fear. In our therapy sessions together, all the members of the family had developed fascinatingly specific and unvaried methods of getting their feelings across while protecting themselves from whatever they were most fearful of. I was the rabble-rouser, constantly campaigning for change and insisting that even if things were good, they could be made better. My father would be the first to take issue with whatever I'd said, and he would argue the longest and the loudest that there was no problem at all. As the arguing between my father and me grew more heated, Lowell's Tourettic twitches would intensify as well. Each time my father and I added another decibel to our accusations and denials, my brother's shouts and kicks would become more wrenching and grotesque in direct proportion.

My brother's symptoms had, in fact, become much worse as a direct result of my diagnosis. Tourette symptoms can, typically, be exacerbated by periods of emotional stress, and the worsening of those symptoms can cause more stress still. In addition, Lowell was struggling to adjust to his having been replaced as the neediest member of the family. Since I had fallen ill, it had come to seem as if my brother and I were engaged in a crude battle for the title of most disadvantaged Handler. In our family therapy sessions, Lowell would be slow to speak, but the agonized expressions on his face, as his body thrashed to the tune of the other's strident shouts, made words seem superfluous to the situation.

Eventually my mother would try to lend some perspective to the impasse that inevitably descended upon me and my father. So softly she would speak. "Murry," she would say, over and over, patting his hand. "Murry, calm down."

When my father ran out of steam, my mother would be surprised to find herself holding center stage. At those moments, I saw my mother's vulnerability as I had never seen it before and have never seen it since. My mother, the assertive mental health professional, in our therapy sessions, would adopt the voice and demeanor of a shy, frightened child. She sacrificed none of her insight or incisiveness. Her views were still carefully considered, her arguments adult and persuasive. But to observe her manner was to peel her life away and sit in the presence of the exposed seed. "May I say something?" was how she would typically begin. Then my mother, who

never needed permission to speak anywhere else, would begin to
skillfully mediate and moderate whatever issue was being debated,
replete with all the apologetic gestures and body language of an
eight-year-old girl admitting that she'd broken the antique vase.

My sister, Lillian, who had generously postponed her wedding as
a result of my illness, and who traveled the farthest to reach Manhattan each week, rarely contributed during the sessions unless it was
requested of her. Somewhat flustered, blushing, and appearing more
uncomfortable than I was used to seeing her, Lillian would often
carefully reemphasize the most compelling points of each argument
being made. Like Switzerland, it seemed that Lillian was most intent
on remaining neutral. More often, though, she would behave as if
she were puzzled by all the fuss. Most of her comments tended to
fall within the realm of "I remember when that happened, but it
never bothered *me*."

I don't know what made me expect anything different outside the
doctor's office, but, for the most part, these were precisely the responses that I got to everything I brought up that day. When I had
finished with my proclamation, my father glanced to either side,
and, with his teeth clenched, said, "Well. If no one else minds, I'd
like to go first."

My father faced me. He took in a long, slow breath and let out
a pained sigh. Then he said, "Look, Evan. I just want you to get
well. That's the bottom line here. Whatever it takes for you to get
well, that's what I'm willing to do. And if what you feel you need
to do to get well is to dump on us, then I'm willing to be dumped
on —"

With that, I threw a fit. I screamed, I whined, I cried and roared
and cursed. I looked to the others in the room, and, as I went from
person to person trying to enlist the help of their memories, their
own pain or shame, their systems of denial and self-protection were
so deeply entrenched that my frustration couldn't completely break

free of my fascination. I found myself alternately crying and laughing. At times, the two overlapped into a kind of otherworldly whimpering hyena's squeal.

I first turned to my sister, who had been a witness to or participant in many of the events I had already laid out. My memory of her was of an extraordinarily talented, angry, withdrawn girl on the verge of womanhood. I remembered the hours and days at a time she would spend locked inside her room, playing her guitar and singing to herself — she had a remarkable musical gift that she would rarely share with anyone else in the family. I clearly recalled the two of us sharing our terror and confusion during the tenser moments of our childhood years, and I was also curious as to how she had dealt with her feelings about Lowell. It was my memory that she had been approached by him in the same ways, for the same services, that I had been. Her responses left me utterly confounded.

"Yeah, I mean, I remember those things, Evan," she said. "Now that you bring them up. But I don't remember them with any of the detail that you seem to. You talk about it as if it all happened yesterday. That was all a long time ago. I don't think about any of those things now."

I just shook my head in amazement, wondering if I was lacking in some component that would have helped me to better shed the weight I felt dragging me down.

"Not ever?" I asked.

"Mmm . . . no. Not really."

"And you don't think that your feelings from those times carried over into anything that came later? Like going to school so far from home; settling down to live somewhere just out of reach; marrying someone whose family and cultural background is as far from ours as you could possibly get?"

Lil kind of chuckled at me, with sympathy and affection, as if I were an extremely endearing lunatic. "I don't really think about why I did those things, Ev. I just did them because that's what I wanted to do. I didn't plan it out."

My mother, who had been silent so far, now leaned forward. When she spoke, there was none of the coy childish demeanor that I had seen in our therapy sessions before. My mother spoke with deep concern, with sorrow, confusion, and with regret.

"Evan," she said. "I didn't know you were in such pain. If I had known, I would have done anything to protect you. But how could we know you were in pain if you didn't ask for help?"

"Mom," I said. "How can you expect an eight-year-old child, who has been rewarded for his independence, for his pretend precociousness, to turn to the adults and say, 'Excuse me, but I'm not really as strong as you've been praising me for being'? The way I got your love and attention was by insisting that I was above it.

"I'm trying to talk about the history of what led us to this place. I think that history may have contributed to what I'm facing, and I know that I need to alter the course of that history in order to get out of this the way I want to. Now, I know that you and Dad have been angry at me. I know you feel you've been slighted, harshly judged, and that I have barricaded myself away from you and hidden behind Jackie. I can sense that you feel a bit usurped by her, and that you're frustrated because I've locked you out of your chance to prove that you're much more capable than I've judged you to be."

I looked around at the four heads that were now bobbing up and down enthusiastically, and I saw that the brightness of recognition was replacing the indignation in their eyes.

"But you've got to try to understand that I believe it's all connected. I feel so trapped into behaving the way I've always behaved, the pattern of sacrificing my own needs to meet someone else's, that I may need to keep you away. I'm afraid that, with you guys too close, I may not do what I need to do to survive. I'll spend the same energy trying to be what I think you want me to be, trying to show you how strong and invincible I am. I can't afford to do that anymore. I'm not bringing these things up today to humiliate you or to get even with you. I'm trying to illustrate to you why I feel that I need to change the ways we respond to each other."

I faced my brother. If there was anyone on this Earth who loved me unconditionally, it was Lowell. Despite whatever wrongs he'd done me long ago, I knew my brother admired me and was devoted to me like no one else ever would be. I knew, and the increase in his symptoms proved clearly, that no one was more shaken by my illness than he was. And, I expected, no one would have been more devastated by my death. Even so, I felt I had to go on.

"Lowell," I said. "A few days ago, you stopped by to see me when you were in the city. You were with me for about an hour, and when I got tired, I asked you to leave. You looked at me as though you were insulted. I love you very much. But it's not always easy to spend time with you. I have to be able to impose some limits, some barriers, because there have been very few in our family relationships. I can't afford to be around anything or anyone that takes energy from me, and, for now, I can't afford to take anyone else's feelings into account. There's too much at stake, and I'm too susceptible to giving myself over in order to spare them."

With that, I started to cry. But this was a different kind of grief than I'd displayed before, and I think that my family saw, for the first time, how vulnerable and lost I really was. While I had insisted on being the leader in my crusade, and while I was still leading the call to arms, this time the enemy I was rallying against was the illusion of my own strength. Sitting with my head bowed, I had at last succeeded in revealing the depths of exhaustion to which my life had led me. When I gathered myself back up, when I felt ready to speak clearly, in a tone that might be seriously considered, I made my points as intently as I could.

"I'm not 'dumping' on anyone," I said softly. "I am trying to talk about things that happened between the people in this room — things that have hurt me. I am trying to get well, yes; and in order to get well, I may need to heal some old injuries — injuries that are sapping some of my strength. For anyone to dismiss this as 'dumping' is wrong. That's not what I'm trying to do here, and it's not what I have done."

I don't know if it was the way I had spoken, or the angle of the tilt of my head, but something about what I'd shown my family must have been startling, because when I looked up, I saw that the irritation that had been etched onto my father's face had softened into a look of troubled concern. In my father's eyes that day, after I was able to relax my need to prove his failings to him, I saw a man who was filled with love for his son, who was frightened of where his life had landed him and who was trying with all his heart to learn what was needed from him. I glanced over to my mother, and I saw a woman who looked stricken by accusations that she wasn't succeeding in helping to save the life of her son, a son she undoubtedly would have sacrificed her own life for. While the force of my initial howl of pain hadn't been enough to penetrate their defenses, something else had happened in my apartment that day. I think the discovery was made that it was not so essential that we all felt the same things, or agreed on the same causes, or shared any of the same beliefs. What was vital was to get behind the family member in need, and support him or her in the way he or she believed would be most helpful. Somehow, during the course of the discussion, a truce was established, and my family and I decided to try to see each other as we were, to hear each other when we spoke, and to slow down our insistence that the others conform to our ideas of what they should be.

In addition, and most important, the simple act of releasing long pent-up emotions allowed me to see the love and generosity that had been in their eyes all along. Although I wasn't able to perceive it that way for some time, the anger I had carried with me as a result of years spent denying my own spirit had seized its own opportunity in the illness. The adolescent rebellion that I had been too adult and mature for as a teenager was simply postponed. As late as it may have come, not only did it set me free from the structure that had previously been strangling me, but that freedom, in turn, then allowed me to reengage with that structure in a more mutually beneficial way. My decision to speak the unspeakable is what ultimately allowed me to permit my struggle to become a group effort — to allow my family to give me the help they were capable of. These are the same principles that go into the making of any good team, whether the game is baseball, basketball, football, cancer, or lacrosse. Each individual must give up the natural drive to distinguish between the glory of his own methods and a teammate's weaknesses. Each needs to contribute to the best of his abilities, to recognize his own strengths and deficiencies, and to give where he can and clear out when he is in the way. The only goal must be to win, a victory for the team. And from that day on, that's what my family started to become.

TRANSCENDENCE

Trips number two and three down the chemotherapy trail proved to be just as exasperating as number one, with the added burden of a lot more physical discomfort. It turned out that Dr. Zweig had been right: I had gotten off easy my first time in the saddle. I'd even go so far as to say, based on the induction course that I had breezed through, that I had no idea what chemotherapy really was. But, as it turned out, I proved to be a quick learner.

We as human beings have a mechanism to defend the body against contamination by bacteria or toxins. It's called vomiting. Not all animals have this ability. It's one of the perks that we get for enduring the power of reason. In this respect, as perhaps in many others, we are all lucky to *be* human beings.

Horses can't vomit. I know this because, when I was a kid, my parents kept a horse at a local stable for my sister. It was a constant source of jealousy. I had no interest in the horse at all, it was just that there was no way they could ever spend as much money on me or a hobby of mine, no matter what I thought of. But I did learn that if a horse eats something that makes it ill, there is a good chance that the horse will die. I don't know what happens to a horse if you give it chemotherapy. Because whatever chemotherapy can do or can't do, whatever it might cure or doesn't, chemotherapy will make you vomit. For hours. For days. For weeks.

It reached a point where there would be nothing unusual about having a violent vomiting attack in the middle of a meal, pausing to catch my breath, and going right back to eating. It became so horrible that I would have laughing fits in the midst of vomiting. Jackie and I would both laugh until we cried, with my grotesque heaves and groans punctuating the giggles and guffaws, and all the sounds melding into marvelous syncopated rhythms. Even after all my treatment was finished, after I was living at home and off all drugs, long out of the hospital, I threw up every day for six months. Not the violent, hour after hour of projectile vomiting caused by the chemotherapy drugs when they were actually in my system. This was a manifestation of some kind of systemic imbalance. A digestive tract and equilibrium completely out of whack, so that, perhaps sitting up quickly in bed; maybe in the shower in the morning; usually with very little warning, I'd wretch and puke. Wretch and puke. Wretch and puke. I wondered if this was going to be a peculiar hygiene problem for years and years to come.

Another of the more compelling problems that arose between these vomit fests during the next hospitalizations had to do with nothing more exotic than my arms. My doctor's decision not to implant a catheter in my chest was beginning to impose its consequences.

My daily schedule of vein puncturings could easily rise above five, and at times climb close to ten. Blood was routinely drawn around dawn for the daily blood tests, as well as any time a blood transfusion was needed (to match the compatibility of the donor blood). Again, blood would be drawn any time a fever appeared, to try to culture the bacteria that was the cause; and when the results of the morning lab tests came back, it was often necessary to administer bottles of fluids and electrolytes to keep the circuits of the body running smoothly. Of course, once the blood products arrived for transfusion, in they went as well, through the same veins in my arms. Until one could no longer be found.

The chemicals that were being passed through my veins were not entirely harmless to them. In fact, they were anything but. The chemotherapy drugs would, quite literally, turn hollow, flexible veins into solid, stiff scar tissue. One by one, the easily seen, easily punctured veins in my arms hardened and dried up. The needles then would be put into my hands. When a vein couldn't be found in my hand, and this was after several attempts at puncturing and rooting around under the skin, then the needle might be placed in my wrist. The soft, inside part of my wrist. For the really unlucky, like I came to be, this happens when they're in urgent need of a blood transfusion, because the thick, cold, maroon glop that makes up a transfusion of packed red blood cells can't travel through just any needle. It requires an extra large needle and often consists of two or more large plastic packages of liquid, which can take more than an hour apiece to drip into the body. If the goo is oozing into a tiny little vein at the inside of the wrist, it *hurts*. It aches with the you-wish-it-were-numbing pain of holding your arm in ice-cold water for too long. For three hours too long. I would hold warm compresses against my arm to try to warm up the liquid flowing in.

Some of the electrolyte chemicals, without which the heart stops beating or the brain's electronic commands can't be followed, have, in concentrated form, a very different alkaline composition from that of the body. This simply means that when dripped in through a vein, these chemicals *sting* like a fire flowing up the length of the inside of the arm. This is how I would spend my days. So, when it was necessary to find a new vein, when an IV line already in place failed to run quickly enough, I would beg and plead to avoid having a new one shoved in. Especially if certain IV nurses were the ones on duty.

Phlebotomy. The insertion of a hollow needle into a viable vein to gain access to the bloodstream. The procedure is performed by phlebotomists. An interesting craft, practiced by an intriguing people. There are degrees of skill, and all the unpredictable ramifications of that fact, in everything. And there are people who are talented at sliding needles into deep, hidden, rolling veins without causing much pain. But of greater importance, much greater importance, there are people who are *untalented* at it. There is a distinct aura, in phlebotomical circles, around certain individuals that are known to be gifted. They can locate veins by lightly running their fingers over the surface of the skin, veins that no one else can see or feel. Like the diviners with their mysterious rods in the desert sands, they can sense the presence of subterranean liquids. Then they'll slide a needle into the channel, quickly, painlessly, with no more fanfare than if they had brushed a stray hair off your forehead. There seems to be a profound relationship in these individuals between their success and their confidence. The "magicians," as they are often called, have complete faith in their abilities to find any vein in any person, no matter how damaged the arm.

The other side of this equation are those whose confidence has been bruised. It is easy to detect a phlebotomist who will fail to find a vein long before the needle touches any skin. You can see the doubt in their eyes. This is why, once a phlebotomist has a bad experience with a patient, the patient is bound to have several bad experiences with that phlebotomist. It's like relief pitching in baseball. There are those pitchers who know that they own the batter, and so they do. Then there are those hitters about whom a pitcher has just a few doubts, and watch him get beat. When my arms were sore and swollen, covered with gruesome bruises; when I was spending my days soaking those arms in warm water to somewhat ease the distress;

when I thought that no one, no one could possibly touch my arm again, ever, without it causing unbearable pain, in would walk the Filipino lady with the falsetto voice. Because she was the worst of all.

The falsetto-voiced Filipino phlebotomist always said the same thing as she walked into my room:

"O-*kay*, Mr. Evans. I have to draw your bloods."

I could hear the apology in her voice. No. There was an apology in the intake of breath before she even spoke. She dreaded this almost as much as I did. She knew she was going to fail before she'd begun.

"O-*kay*, Mr. Evans. Which arm today?"

My veins could sense her hesitation. Veins have their own peculiar survival technique in that they can actually retreat and hide. I don't know if it's a documented medical phenomenon, but I've seen it happen. Few things in this world are more ruthless than bad veins that can smell a phlebotomist's fear. As soon as the flat, falsetto tone of her voice reached my ears, I'd feel my veins constrict and shrink deeper under my skin. You could almost hear them chuckling. They would play with her while I writhed in agony.

As soon as the tourniquet was pulled tightly around my scrawny bicep, my whole arm, already sore and swollen, would begin to throb and turn bright red.

"O-*kay*, Mr. Evans. Hold still."

I knew there wasn't a blind man's chance in Hell that she was going to get a vein. She knew before she had dinner last night that she wasn't going to get a needle in my vein today.

"O-*kay*, Mr. Evans. Little pinch."

Little pinch, my bony, malnourished ass. The needle was in my flesh, and the pain shot up the inside of my arm and wrapped itself around my neck like a six-foot rough woolen scarf. It wound itself around the base of every dormant hair follicle, then spread out over my scalp and coated it with a hot poultice of sharp needles.

"Hold still, Mr. Evans."

94

At least she didn't say "o-*kay*" this time.

I had learned a preference early on that, I guess, made me different from most of the other patients. First of all, when a needle does hit a vein, when it slides successfully *into* the vein, there is no pain. Almost none at all. So I usually knew before the nurse whether we'd gotten a hit or not. And to me, there was no torture worse than someone rooting around and digging in my flesh to find a vein that they had missed on the way in. I don't think anyone ever found a vein this way on me anyway. So I would say, as soon as the miss became apparent, "Hey. Hey, hey, HEY! Hold it. Just . . . just . . . okay, STOP! Look, I'd much rather you take the needle out completely and start all over with a fresh stick than move the needle around while it's already in my skin." And, of course, they all took this to mean that I was a masochist and really loved pain. Who else would want to be stuck again?

But I knew that if the needle went in the right place the next time, there'd be no pain. And if the needle didn't go in right the next time, and didn't go in right the time after that . . . then, *then* the falsetto-ed vampiress would say, "O-*kay*, Mr. Evans, I send somebody else in."

Now *that* was "O-*kay*"!

You see, the policy was, three strikes and you're out. If you endured three stabs, and no blood poured forth, then they would endure the delays entailed by calling in the other IV nurse on the floor. If you'd really been suffering, and all the nurses were afraid to try, they'd bring in one of the magicians, from wherever in the hospital he or she might be. What a sight that was, to see one of those blessed surveyors of the internal aqueducts glide — no, float — into the room. My muscles would relax, my heart would slow down, and my veins, my precious, perverse veins, would swell with blood and float up to the surface, ready to meet the needle.

*   *   *

The other plague that struck me hard and wouldn't let go was a constant barrage of rashes. I came to understand that I am as supersensitive to drugs and chemicals that I come in contact with as the most delicate of endangered wildlife are to changes in their habitats.

Before chemotherapy drugs are administered there is another drug to be taken, allopurinol, which is given to help the body deal with the byproducts of all the cells that will soon be dying off inside. I proved to be allergic to this drug. Each time it was administered I broke out in a ferocious red rash that started immediately below my neck and ended at my ankle. As this rash began to fade, about two weeks later, I might be put on an antibiotic that would again cause my flesh to explode. To blossom, with all the brilliance of rolling hills of wild flowers. Again and again I turned into a contoured topographical map of the substances that were being run through me. I would look at my skin, at my body, and the disfiguration was so extreme that it was hard to imagine that it could ever smooth out. Even if the rashes were to leave, I couldn't envision that stretched, ravaged wrapping paper ever fitting right again.

After the second round of treatment was finished, I was sent home to rest for another month before the final dose. A few days after getting home, though, my skin erupted once more. Despite the fact that I was currently taking no drugs, I was being seized by some force that was crimping and wrinkling my skin in a fiery pageant of colors and patterns. I haven't used the word "itch" yet, only because it is dreadfully inadequate. There is a level of itching that goes beyond itching and becomes a grotesque pain that *includes* itching. Then it becomes a torture that will bend your mind. It can even become so consuming that it is very easy to injure yourself, with the deluded notion that the itching might be quieted. I, myself, had to be talked out of raking a fork over my arms. I thought that perhaps, if I could scrape the rash off, my skin would then heal over and the rash would be gone. It would have been so much more bearable to be one giant scab than to itch for one more instant.

Besides the suffering, we were worried. What was causing this rash? I made an appointment to see Dr. Zweig.

If anything could compete with the horror of life on the floor at Sloan-Kettering, it was the outpatient clinic. The only way to procure a visitation with one's attending physician at that hospital, short of checking oneself in, was to make an appointment for one of the two weekly "clinic days" each doctor conducted. The clinic was crowded and noisy, with people in all stages of recovery and deterioration, and the difference between my appointment time and when I actually saw a doctor was consistently in the two- to four-hour range. This time was spent sitting in the giant waiting room while the PA system droned incessantly with mispronounced name after mispronounced name.

"*My*-ran-da . . . Miran . . . *My*-ran-da Thhhowmaas. Vin . . . Vine . . . Vine-seent Wojell. Vojel. Vo-*gel*? Vine-ceent Vogel. Eh-vahn . . . E-Evonne . . . Evonne Huyn-del." That was me. The names were called by the technicians in the blood lab, which was my first stop after the waiting room. Hours later, if the doctor determined that more blood tests were needed, I then went back to waiting until some other version of my name was called again. It would usually be startlingly different from the one announced two or three hours earlier. If a blood transfusion proved necessary I went back to the blood lab to get my blood drawn once more, to be tested for donor compatibility, then waited another two hours for the blood to be ordered and delivered from the blood bank. *Then* I went to the transfusion room to be drugged and transfused, which could take anywhere from one to six hours itself. This could easily stretch into a twelve-hour day. And I shared this routine with hundreds of other sick people, three days a week for weeks on end. I usually felt I could barely survive this ordeal, and I was twenty-four years old. How anyone sixty, seventy, eighty years old could possibly endure was a mystery to me.

My way of navigating these treacherous waters was to become, for the first time in my life, a criminal of sorts. I knew that there was another blood lab, on another floor, intended for use only for the blood drawn from inpatients of the hospital. Since the authorization slips used to instruct that lab were identical to those used in the outpatient clinic, I would check into the clinic, take one of the blood forms, forge the doctor's signature, and take it to the other blood lab. There, though I'd get some funny looks, I would get the technicians to draw my blood, run the tests quickly, and hand me the results. If the blood count results were what I knew they should be and I had no other immediate complaints, I'd skip the doctor visit and I'd leave. I'd go home. If the results indicated that I would need a transfusion, I'd go back up to the clinic and pester the doctors and nurses dashing from room to room until I got one of them to stop and write out the orders for the transfusion blood. That way, by the time I got in to see the doctor for my official appointment, the blood would be arriving at the transfusion room, where I would be sent to receive it. This is how I would cut out three or four hours from my day. Three or four hours of sitting in a giant room with two hundred other sick people, waiting for a doctor to take me into a room and read the same numbers that I read off the computer printout myself.

At times I would wonder if I might be contributing to some of the problems of the hospital by doing this. Was I compromising someone else's care by manipulating the system this way? I didn't let those thoughts bother me for very long. I saw myself as I imagined my ancestors must have been, vying for a job on the food line of a concentration camp. That stolen carrot, those two extra crusts of bread, could mean the difference between life and death. I saw my time, those precious two hours, three hours, of time, and the energy that went into them — for resting; for making love; for living —

as every bit as essential to my survival as those scraps of food. So I became a thief. I collected stolen moments, in the hope they might add up to an extra day, an extra week, until the liberation.

When I finally got in to see Zweig on that particular day, he was even more distracted and dismissive than usual.

"This is what you came in about?" he said. "This? This? It's a rash!"

"I know it's a rash. But it came out of nowhere. And I've got a fever. I got the rash and a low-grade fever at the same time."

"What's your temperature?"

"About a hundred."

"A hundred? A hundred and what? I thought you said you had a fever!"

It's amazing what fear can make you put up with. Fear and ignorance, neither of which I was used to being the victim of. I didn't know at the time that a drug rash can occur days, or even weeks, after a patient has completely stopped taking a medication. I learned it that day, though. And I also didn't know that a frightened, sick young man and his family don't have to be grateful for the abusive attentions of a troubled man, no matter what kind of an M.D. he holds or how prized is his specialty. But Dr. Zweig taught me that, too. And now that I had learned my lessons, it was time to find myself a doctor who hadn't developed what appeared to be such a deep hatred of the people needing his help.

Not that anyone at that hospital was going to make it easy. I scheduled an appointment to meet for a consultation with a Dr. Elizabeth Klaus. If my visions of myself as a reincarnated Jew fighting persecution by vicious Nazis in an elaborate scheme for my destruction needed any reinforcement, Elizabeth Klaus was the perfect choice to help.

Dr. Klaus was a hefty woman who spoke with a thick German accent, and whose voice rasped as the result of a deeply committed relationship with a pack of cigarettes, which I rarely saw her without.

I don't know why they were visible; the doctors' coats had pockets. But she would routinely either have them in her hand when she entered a room or take them out of her pocket and place them, with her keys, on the table between us. It was as if she was making a defiant proclamation. "Here, Cancer Patient. See the doctor. She has no fear!"

I was being coached, through all of this, by the psychiatrist that I was seeing, Dr. Yehuda Nir. As a result of his own experience at Sloan-Kettering, Dr. Nir had already proven invaluable with his advice on how to best handle the inflated egos of the doctors and how to gain access to the few advantages of the hierarchical systems of the hospital. In shopping for a new doctor, I was warned, beware.

"They will love to hear everything bad you have to say about Zweig," Dr. Nir advised me. "They will want all the dirt, so they can use it for themselves later. Then, they will turn on you. Once they hear what you have to say, they will do everything they can to protect him and to punish you for attacking him. Say nothing but 'Dr. Zweig and I have different ways of communicating, and I find it difficult to talk with him. I need a doctor whom I can communicate with.' "

"But how can I find a doctor that I like if I don't really tell them what I'm looking for? I want someone who will understand all the other things that I'm doing. The healings, nutrition, the —"

"You won't find it there. You find a way to use them as best you can. You will know if you've found a doctor you can use. You don't have to tell them about yourself. They can't handle it."

Inside I laughed at Dr. Nir. We had begun to work together only about three months earlier, but I was already impressed with the way his estimation of his fellow humans consistently fell well below my own. I think Yehuda Nir was the first person I ever met that I could describe as being more suspicious and jaded than myself. But one of the problems I was having in my therapy, in trying to view the world as a less hostile environment, had a lot to do with how often his bleak view seemed to be right on target.

At my consultation with Elizabeth Klaus it was as if my shrink had written the script. First, she wanted to know if I'd told Zweig that I was seeing her. I told her that I hadn't, that at that point it didn't seem necessary. Then she wanted to hear every complaint that I had about him. She pried, she schmoozed, she coaxed, and she joked. She smiled knowingly and told me she understood how hard it could be. I stuck to my story: we have trouble communicating.

"What kind of trouble?" she asked. "I can't help you if you don't tell me what the problem is."

It had become a battle of wills, it seemed. It was too perfect. I thought I must be creating this scenario out of my own expectations. My therapist had prepared me to anticipate defeat, and that was what I had brought upon myself. I decided to break character and give her a chance. I pulled back the veil a quarter of an inch and let her in. No sooner had I shared with her one of the many instances of Zweig's insensitivity than Elizabeth Klaus cut me off and said, "Well, that's just ridiculous. Dr. Zweig is a fine doctor, and I don't see what the problem could be. I think that you're going through a very difficult time, I can see by your chart that you're not doing as well as you were a couple of months ago, and I think that you're overreacting. There's no need to take out your troubles on Dr. Zweig."

I sat very still and I stared at Elizabeth Klaus. I sat no more than eighteen inches away from her, but I allowed myself to examine her as if she were not a person but a specimen. Time seemed to slow down around me, while my mind raced and I pondered my next move. Then, the little voice inside my head that keeps me company all day long started talking. The voice said, "If you ever try to tell anyone about this, they'll never believe you. They'll think you've become completely paranoid. If anyone ever told *you* about this, you wouldn't believe *them*. I'm here, right here where it's happening, and I can't believe it."

The next day, my phone rang at home. It was Dr. Zweig. He demanded to know why I had met with Elizabeth Klaus. Not only was I surprised that my visit with her hadn't been protected by a rather honored regulation known as doctor/patient confidentiality, but I also quickly gleaned that Zweig was enraged. He launched into a monologue that I listened to in wonder.

"I mean, okay, you had a rash. You had a rash, and if I didn't give you, uh, the uh, the proper amount of sympathy to please you, well, I . . . I apologize for that. I suppose. Although I don't know what I'm supposed to do about a rash, anyway. I mean, we'll . . . we'll . . . we'll get you a prescription, if that's what you want. But nowadays it's just, well, obviously, it's always the doctor's fault. I mean, I accept that. With all the malpractice suits going on now, well . . . the doctor is always the monster. That's the way it seems to be, and I'll just have to live with that. Because, okay, okay, the patient dies. So? So? That makes me a monster? The patient died. If that makes me a monster, so be it. I just want you to know that I'm still willing to treat you. I've thought about it and I've decided that I'm still perfectly willing to remain as your physician. The fact that you consulted with another doctor . . . nothing that has transpired will alter my ability to treat you."

"EXCEPT YOUR FUCKING *INSANITY!*" I wanted to yell. I couldn't see how anyone who was not losing his mind could find it remotely appropriate to phone a twenty-four-year-old man in grave danger of dying of leukemia and plead for sympathy about some other patient who had died. A man earning, probably, over two hundred thousand dollars a year; who leaves his patients in the hospital each night, alone, while he goes home to his wife, or his lover, or whomever he chooses; who chooses, once again, the next morning, to return to the hospital, or to quit, or to go into advertising, or whatever he wants to do! Who has his health, and therefore all the freedom anyone could ever wish to have. He called me on the phone and told me that he was still willing to be my physician.

I remembered the way my father had looked after his first phone conversation with Dr. Zweig. I could feel my body shrinking into the same submissive pose. I was sitting on the floor of my apartment, trembling, with tears running down my face. But I summoned up all my courage, and, borrowing my father's deceptively controlled telephone voice, I spoke for both of us. I said, "I appreciate that, Dr. Zweig. I would like you to continue. I will continue to see you in the clinic for the next two weeks while I continue to meet with other doctors. When I make my decision as to who my new doctor will be, then I will let you know and you can arrange to have my records transferred to them."

"Okay, Mr. Handler. I'll see you in clinic then." And he was off the phone.

I found a new doctor quickly, and though we still saw each other often, in and around the hospital, I never exchanged another word with Dr. Leonard Zweig.

And I never did get anything for that rash.

*   *   *

As I prepared to enter the hospital for the third, and final, round of chemotherapy, I was armed with a new doctor, and an excitement that came from the feeling that the end of the nightmare was near. My new doctor was Jesselyn Melman, a woman who wore a soft cushion of friendliness over her otherwise officious demeanor. Compared with Zweig and some of the others I had met so far, Dr. Melman seemed like a blessing sent from heaven.

During the previous two months my mother had continued to gather all kinds of information about other treatment centers in this country. In fact, my parents had both succeeded, in spite of my constant efforts to find fault with and exclude them, at finding many ways to be truly helpful. Not only had they continued to maintain their stalwart schedule to meet my everyday needs — by bringing me food when I was in the hospital and endlessly shopping for me and laundering the seven sets of bedclothes I sweated through nightly — but they had also put together the Evan Handler Recovery Fund, the organization overseen by my aunt and a family friend that solicited donations to offset my living expenses while I remained unable to support myself. Also within the fund's domain were the medical costs that outdistanced my extensive, yet still insufficient, insurance coverage. With a steady stream of friends, business associates, and relatives, my parents had continued to keep the blood-donor room jumping as well, making sure that for every pint withdrawn for me, at least a quart was put back in.

In an even more extraordinary development, they had begun to distribute a newsletter describing my progress as well as the stresses they were under. Whoever called them at home, during the few hours they had to rest themselves, was thanked for their concern and put on the mailing list. While a few old friends mentioned this newsletter to me with narrowed eyes that suggested their suspicion that my parents were cracking under the strain, I saw it as a brilliant device. The exhaustion that is unavoidable to parents of a sick child, even an adult child, is enough to overwhelm the strongest individual. The hidden demands, one of which is the exertion of energy necessary to respond to people's well-meant and desired inquiries and good wishes, can be the straw that breaks their backs. When some of the well-wishers' eyes glaze over, in a clear indication that they really never intended their offers of compassion to be seized, the heart can break as well. My parents were simply accepting the offers coming forth and sharing their burden in a fashion that didn't increase their already superhuman load. By revealing themselves in the newsletter, both the good news and the bad, they gave their friends the option of tuning in or tuning out, without having to suffer the indignity of facing those who could not cope with what my parents dealt with daily.

Amongst the information my mother had gathered were often conflicting reports of what was the best course of treatment for someone in my position. All the experts had their own opinions, and many of them would warn against using anyone's advice other than their own. Others, though, might be quite gracious, and simply say that there were drastically differing opinions on the matter. This information, while very helpful and necessary to wade through, could lead to agonizing decisions. For instance, I learned through my mother that doctors at one highly respected hospital had told her that there was no evidence to support there being any benefit from having a third round of chemotherapy. No one had been able to demonstrate that another tour through Hell would actually have an effect on my chances for long-term survival.

I brought this up to my new doctor. She said, "Yes, Evan. It's true. But while we can't say for sure that it is beneficial for you to have more treatment, we think that it probably is, and so we recommend it."

What was I supposed to do with that? We were talking about a month-long ordeal, which, by itself, had a 10 percent chance of killing me. How was I supposed to enter into that with the knowledge that it might not be necessary and I'd have the same chance for recovery without it? I had no idea what to do.

In the moments that I had been able to sleep between the fevers, the medications, and the blood transfusions that made no distinction between night and day, I was gripped and transported by furious dream activity beyond anything I had experienced before. During my first week in the hospital, I had repeatedly had the dream that I was in prison, sharing a cell with a dangerous inmate. I had been accused of killing someone by stabbing them through the eye with a ballpoint pen. I knew I hadn't done it, but I had to endure the situation and survive, until I got my day in court. When my day for justice arrived I strode into the courtroom, eager to reclaim my freedom, only to stare in horror as I was shown a film of myself committing the crime. I had that dream every night for a week.

During the second hospital stay, I'd had a dream in which I was chewing on long metal nails and shards of glass. There was no pain involved, only a squeamish sensation as the sharp objects were driven by my own jaws deep, deep into the flesh of my gums. My left upper gum, specifically. A few days later, a serious infection was caused by an impacted wisdom tooth in that very spot.

Then, as the third hospitalization approached, as I was faced with the decision of how to best proceed with my medical treatment, I had the epic dream of my life. I found myself in a hellish, medically themed production of *Hamlet.* Not only was the play that I dreamt about perfectly symbolic of the terrible indecision that I was suffering through, but I also found myself unfamiliar with my lines and my surroundings. I'd wind up lost, cornered by enormous stage flats that conspired to trap me in inescapable configurations; other actors chased me around with machetes as I tried to escape, stumbling over the webs of IV tubing and medicine bottles dangling down from between my legs. At the play's intermission, I was told that I was being replaced in the next act by another actor. The ultimate indignity, though, was still to come. As I heard the second act beginning without me, and as I searched for an exit from the building, from the whole humiliating nightmare, I was stopped backstage, and asked to contribute money for the cast party.

Once outside the building, I found myself wandering on a wet country road, where I was approached by Jackie. Jackie pulled close and told me that she had a message for me from Steven, an actor friend who had, himself, had cancer as a teenager. Jackie told me, in the dream, that the way to "get home" was the same way that Steven had done it. The key was in his hitchhiking technique. Walk along the road, I was told, and let two cars pass. Then, turn and face the third.

I checked back into Sloan-Kettering and I did it all again.

R & R

Temescal Canyon sits in the highlands overlooking the Pacific Ocean just north of Los Angeles, in Pacific Palisades, California. Back from the main road, in the midst of a state nature preserve, is the Presbyterian Church Retreat; a ramshackle collection of meeting houses, cafeteria, and dirty, miniature, summer camp–type bunkhouses. This is where, for one week each month, Carl Simonton and his staff conduct the workshops of the Simonton Cancer Center.

Jackie and I arrived in early March for a week of therapy sessions, instruction in guided imagery, words of wisdom from Dr. Simonton himself, and we didn't know what else. Not long after we'd dropped our bags onto the gritty floor of our sparsely furnished, screened-in cabin, we started to hear about the fire walk. No one would say much about it, at first. We were told we'd have to wait and see. But we were promised a belief-altering thrill when the week's activities culminated in a demonstration of the mind-over-matter miracle of walking through a fifteen-foot channel of hot coals without suffering injury.

I glanced suspiciously at the other seminar participants. They were a collection of Caucasian adults, all but me between the ages of thirty-five and seventy, none looking too robust or healthy. There was a woman in her sixties with bone cancer who walked with a cane, and a woman in her thirties with nearly translucent skin who wore a jet-black wig that sat crookedly on her head. All day long I'd watch her tug at it, each yank bringing it too far over one ear or the other, somehow never hitting the middle mark. There was the woman from Alaska with enormous breasts who told us the first day that she'd just had her second one removed, and the sprightly old Irish munchkin man dying of liver cancer who sipped whiskey from a flask all day. I had just gotten out of the hospital one week before myself, after being inside for the better part of the past six months. My muscles were so weak that standing upright and taking ten steps felt like walking a mile on stilts. I was drawn back to the voice of the staff member speaking as we were told that, at the end of the demonstration, we would each have our own opportunity to blow our minds even more by taking the fiery walk ourselves.

Wonderful, I thought.

As soon as the fire walk subplot had been established, the meetings began. There was a group of several instructor/therapists, each with his or her own brand of New Age, psychoinspirational speaking, each trying to illustrate various points of Simonton's philosophies. In between these seminars and workshops, we would be entitled to spend three half-hour sessions with our assigned therapist, with more available for a negotiated price. Then we were told about the various kinds of massage therapies available to us over the course of the session. We were encouraged to take full advantage of the incredible healing talents of the body-work professionals joining us for the week, and it was recommended that we try them all by having at least one massage a day — costing only forty dollars apiece.

I had paid two thousand one hundred dollars "tuition" to attend the Simonton Cancer Center. Jackie, as my "support person," had paid somewhat less, to cover her food and lodging, and this was all in addition to our cross-country airfare. It had been a fear of mine all along — indeed, through the whole illness, with my various healers — that I might be just one more desperate soul feeding the hungry hands of opportunistic con artists. When, after each of the first three workshops, we were offered audiotapes, *for sale,* by whichever individual had conducted the seminar — tapes for relaxation, for pain release, for childhood regression, tapes on trust — I was ready to storm out and demand my money back. When I forced myself, through my nervousness, to mention my complaint to one of the instructors, I was told that it would probably be a good topic to bring up in my individual therapy. Since I had a session scheduled for later that day, I decided to hang in a little longer and seek some satisfaction before taking off.

Barbi Monde was a youngish blond woman who could have served as a model for those who like to ridicule Southern California's penchant for wide-eyed cheerfulness, and breathy, awestruck spirituality. In a match made anywhere but Heaven, Barbi was assigned to me as my personal therapist.

"Isn't that in-ter-est-cen, Evan?" Barbi said, fascinated. She pronounced the word using four syllables and ending with the common West Coast substitution of *-een* for *-ing.* "What do you think it is about your relationship to money that makes you so angry about spend-*een* it on yourself?"

Baffled, I took a moment to get my thoughts together. "I don't have any problem spending money on myself," I said. "I have a problem with arriving someplace that I've had to borrow money to afford, only to discover that a large portion of the recommended experience isn't covered in that fee. I think everything should be included in the "tuition" price, or else it should be clear in advance that many of the tools and activities are an extra cost."

Barbi gently took the small spiral notebook I was fidgeting with from my hands. Wearing a joyful smile, the kind you use when you're about to give someone a wonderfully generous and unexpected gift, she wrote in a large, neat script. Barbi handed me back my book, smiling even wider than before. As I read her words, I could feel the heat radiating from her glowing satisfaction with herself. She was apparently intoxicated by her ability to impart wisdom and relieve the suffering of others. Barbi had written,

Things are never the way they seem.
There is good in everything. Always be grateful.

When I looked back up at her, Barbi's smile was stretched so wide I thought her face might split apart to reveal the coils and wires and transistors I suspected were buried beneath. When she had finished saying a silent prayer for my recovery, Barbi's eyes popped open and she chimed, "Well, that's the end of our first session!"

Somehow, that made me laugh. I laughed very hard, and it went on for a long time. At first, Barbi seemed frightened. She didn't know me, and it was obvious that she had no idea what I was laughing about. But it only took a moment for her "feel good about everything" instincts to kick back in, and soon Barbi was laughing along with me, smiling and nodding in agreement, as if we were actually sharing the same joke.

To me, it was clear that I had escaped from one lunatic asylum, only to enroll myself in another. I decided to stay, just to see what might happen. If nothing else, it promised to be a good show, and at twenty-one hundred dollars admission, I wasn't keen on missing any of the action.

In spite of her initial resistance in recognizing my complaint, Barbi soon made it clear that she was determined to get me a little something extra on my trip to California. In the course of conversation she became aware of my interest in Louise Hay, a woman who had become well known as a healer and spiritual leader, largely through her newly popularized book *You Can Heal Your Life*. Louise was the healer who'd helped my friend Steven through his illness as a teenager, and, though he had tried to interest her in my plight, she had been too busy to take on any new clients. Barbi helped run some of Louise's weekly get-togethers, and she agreed to take me along to one during the week.

I was, at first, confused by Barbi's secretiveness about our field trip. She had sternly insisted that I tell no one else at the center of our plans, which I could somewhat understand in terms of avoiding the impression that I was receiving preferential treatment. But, in addition, Barbi would not reveal what nights of the week Louise's group would meet, or which meeting we would attend. When I tried to press her, or, as the week wore on, when I tried to get some reassurance that our plans were still intact, Barbi would gush with a lot of talk about which group was the best to visit; about how difficult it was to know whether Louise would actually appear or not; about a host of veiled, obtuse mumblings that made little sense to me. On Thursday, at lunch in the cafeteria, Barbi strode by me with a peculiarly stricken look on her face. It wasn't until she had passed and was out of my field of vision that I realized she had spoken. Her words hung in her wake, taking a moment to penetrate my confusion.

"Meet me in the parking lot at eight o'clock tonight."

I turned to respond, but Barbi was already sitting across the room with the staff. She was leaning forward, engrossed in conversation, seemingly oblivious to me, giving no indication that we had communicated at all. I had no idea what all the espionage was about, but I finally felt like I was getting my money's worth.

"Now, Evan," Barbi was saying, after hurrying me into her car in the dark of the unpaved parking lot. "I'm going to ask you to scootch down under the seat until we're out on the road."

Barbi was reaching down under my feet to clear out the debris that was carpeting the floor of her car. She spoke as she threw fistfuls of wadded up papers and crushed diet soda cans into the back seat. I had irrepressible flashback memories of the puzzling excitement I had felt when riding in the car of one of my schoolteachers. The pride that accompanied the invitation into the teacher's private sanctum was demolished by the evidence of their untidy mortal habits. While I crouched low in the foot well beneath the passenger seat, Barbi drove roughly over the bumpy dirt road toward the Pacific Coast Highway. The last time I'd been smuggled anywhere was in high school, riding in the trunk with two other friends trying to avoid paying for a drive-in movie. Never before, though, had I been forced to sneak *away* from any place.

Barbi calmed down, a bit, once we were on the road. During the short drive into Santa Monica, sitting back up in the car seat, I learned the reason for her nervousness.

"Carl wouldn't like it if he knew," she said.

"Wouldn't like what?" I asked. "Is it that he doesn't want the clients leaving the compound? Or he doesn't like the staff fraternizing with the inmates? What?"

"He'd be mad if he knew I was taking you to see Louise."

Ahhh. Professional alternative-therapy jealousy. I was being secretly whisked away to an enemy rally, my mind primed for subversion back home. I was stunned. This would have been my very last guess at an explanation.

I had, in fact, found Carl Simonton to be a fascinating and admirable man. He appeared to be in his mid- to late forties, with a rather dour-looking, bearded face. Carl dressed simply, in casual, country clothes — usually jeans and a flannel shirt — and he spoke directly and compellingly. In opposition to his appearance, he was irreverent, and he was funny. His lectures focused on the themes of his book, and then reached beyond. He spoke of the importance of living a life that was in tune with one's chosen purpose, and he had developed effective methods for exploring what that might be. In addition to the somewhat esoteric techniques of meditation and imagery he imparted, Simonton had gone further and designed concrete methods for people to plan how to put their choices into practice. In this vein, he encouraged all the seminar participants to design a "six-month plan," in which they would set realistic goals toward guiding their lives in the direction of their desire. As Joseph Campbell advises his readers to "follow your own bliss," Carl Simonton would often intone, "The path of least resistance is the way of greatest joy."

The entire session in Temescal Canyon, in fact, had been well designed, and after my initial anger, I had been drawn into an embracing of the experience. One lecture of Carl's led to another instructor's more practical workshop, which in turn laid the groundwork for another of Carl's inspirational sermons. Whatever his own abilities or difficulties, he was able to convey a great enthusiasm for life, and for insisting on living it on one's own terms — whether free from illness, or saddled with a myriad of ailments. Carl seemed especially proud of the story of his arrival in California years before. Late for an appointment, behind in his work, he insisted on being driven first to the beach, where he put together his kite and flew it in the wind blowing off the Pacific Ocean. Carl loved to fly his kite, you see, and so it was his first priority in life. Once he had experienced the pleasure he was able to provide himself, the pleasure that the world made available to him, then Carl was ready to go to work. What I was even more impressed with, above all else, was his lack of pretension. Carl seemed to believe what he was teaching, and he seemed to teach it because he believed it. His lack of self-promotion and self-congratulation didn't prepare me for Barbi's description of a man who was plagued by the relative obscurity of his pioneering work.

I wrote it off as another illustration of the mysterious wisdom in Barbi's first cryptic message to me: "Things are never the way they seem." Then, in the thickly carpeted living room where Louise Hay's support group was meeting, I tried to remember the rest of her advice: "There is good in everything. Always be grateful."

If you've ever seen a tall, blond woman with intense, unapologetic eyes glaring out at you from a television talk show while unabashedly embracing a child's stuffed animal, you may very well have been introduced to Louise Hay.

Louise spoke with a deep voice she used to impart a practiced sense of commanding calm and spiritual connectedness. She was sitting in front of a fireplace mantel, surrounded by a large group of mostly young people who sprawled across the living room, across the furniture; who spread themselves like paste into every nook and crevice of the room. Eager faces, some grinning, some teary-eyed, all painted with a blend of expressions seen wherever pained souls seek communal reassurance. A touching mixture of the joyous relief that comes from finding a refuge of like-minded wanderers, and a tentative hesitancy to reveal too much — lest they be rejected here like they have come to expect everywhere else. Most of the young adults were holding, caressing, snuggling one or more of the dozens of stuffed animals sitting amongst them. One by one, they offered updates to Louise and the group about their problems, their hopes, their bank accounts, and their health. They spoke of sexual abuse by stepfathers, addiction to unhealthy lovers, and about the number of T cells left in their bloodstreams. All seemed convinced, as Louise espoused, that the universe was structured to provide all that was needed to any who were ready to receive it. If you were lacking something necessary to your happiness, the answer lay in why you were keeping higher powers from providing you with what you claimed to desire.

"You know, Louise, I have been talking, week after week, about my screenplay."

It was Bill speaking. Bill was a slim man with close-cropped sandy hair who spoke with the barely contained distress of an unfortunate choice for a *Candid Camera* stunt. His manner was reminiscent of the overly earnest victims who had to be rescued by Allen Funt before they collapsed into tears, too distraught to be viewed further by a family audience.

"Now I understand that my relationship to my father has kept me from feeling that I deserve any kind of success," Bill was saying. "I realize that I have tried to please him by remaining the failure that he expects me to be. But I have been doing my affirmations in the mirror every day. I have told Jason that he has to move out, because I know I need a lover who believes in me as much as I believe in myself. I really know in my heart that I am a good writer, and I am sure that I am going to sell my screenplay. I even have a figure that I've been visualizing. Eighty thousand dollars. I know that I am going to sell my screenplay for eighty thousand dollars. So, if I am doing my affirmations; if I believe that I deserve success; if I know that I am ready to accept success into my life, why isn't it happening?"

I already had confusing, mixed feelings about Louise Hay's philosophies. I looked to her books and tapes for the same comfort and inspiration as the others in the room with me — and I found plenty of it. Louise was a survivor of serious illness herself, and many of her ideas had been incorporated into my own emerging amalgamation of techniques. For instance, I could easily imagine that someone's reluctance to confront specific obstacles in his life might inhibit his drive to get well. It seemed reasonable to me to investigate if my illness was protecting me from anything and, if so, to wrestle with those fearful issues. This practice fell into the category of grabbing control and influence where it might be available — again, to gain the *greatest potential* for success. And the room wasn't empty of positive examples. A lot of what I saw and heard that night were miraculous accounts of love and will conquering fear and circumstance. People who had been pounded by life, but never into submission. People who insisted on scouring the terrain of every misfortune for a foothold, any aspect of it that might be turned into some form of opportunity. Where I started to lose my connection to Louise's work, just like that of most of her peers with whom I was familiar, was when they promoted their philosophies as formulas. Theories that I found invaluable for increasing my conceivable influence over my illness were being seized on by others at the meeting as concrete equations, and those people were not being corrected. As helpful as I found some of the talk in the room, at times I found the discussion swirling around me to be grotesque and dangerous.

Louise's groups had expanded to several evenings a week after the explosion of the AIDS crisis. Awareness of the epidemic was multiplying exponentially during the spring of 1986, when I visited California, and it formed a strong undercurrent to a lot of the searching going on that night in Santa Monica. It is logical to wonder, when trying to wrest some reassurance that the world is a safe, protective place, about a virus that kills indiscriminately and ruthlessly. This was the type of dilemma that made it impossible for me to agree with the more trusting, faith-oriented aspects of Louise's, or anyone's, beliefs. While I found value in asking myself how I might benefit from my illness — how I could use it to improve my life once the danger had passed — I cringed when I heard people distort this kind of eagerness to improve into questions of why certain groups had brought disasters upon themselves. There was some talk of how homosexual men had needed to confront the self-hatred that kept them closeted and their inability to love as symbolized by promiscuous sexuality, and so had somehow manufactured the virus as a means of accomplishing this positive evolutionary step. When many in the group later began wondering aloud why the Ethiopians needed the famine that was starving their nation, why they had brought it upon themselves, I was staggered by the absence of a ringing denunciation.

There is a distinct difference between committing oneself to using a crisis for growth and improvement and deciding that those changes are the reason why the crisis occurred. I said many times during the week spent at the Simonton Center, "If leukemia doesn't kill me, I'll probably live a better life as a result of having had it." But that didn't stop me from viewing the entire era as an abomination. Never once have I been glad it happened to me. Nor have I ever felt that it was something that I needed or something that was as it should have been.

Louise ended the meeting as I had hoped she would, with a series of hands-on healings. This was the aspect of the meeting, of the whole holistic healing movement, that I found most thrilling. The notion of human beings offering the power of their own souls to another in need; the transference of the gift of life force from one individual to another, was something that I found mesmerizing. I suppose it is the only blind faith that I have ever allowed myself to indulge in. While I prayed often in times of danger, I never felt certain there was anyone who heard. But in Louise Hay's living room I could feel her hands on my shoulders and chest. I could look up from my position on the floor to see the fifty or sixty other people, each touching another, making a human chain to the point where one of them touched Louise. I experienced a rejuvenating rush of strength as this undeniably powerful woman willed the energy of the entire room into my body. This was, for me, the apex of my journey so far. The culmination of months spent trying to convince myself that human beings possess the ability to create the circumstances they crave and that others can help them to conquer the forces teamed against them. That the world is full of miracles and that a miracle was available to me. I rose up off the floor intoxicated with my willingness to open myself up to the goodness available in the room, even when I disagreed so feverishly with much of what was said. I nearly floated back to Barbi's side, so sure of my destiny; so worried that time might come to mock me by proving me a fool.

I left Louise chuckling to myself at what I thought of as the silliness of her parting advice. As I said good-bye and angled for the door, Louise warned me of the power of color in affecting people's outlook and potential. She cautioned me about the muting qualities of black clothing, and recommended that I wear colors such as green and blue, which symbolized growth and life — the colors associated with the water and the plants of planet Earth. I thanked Louise profusely, and headed out the door. I had been aware of her beliefs before heading over to her house that night, yet I had chosen, in spite of them, to wear my favorite sweatshirt to the meeting. It was made of heavy jet-black cotton, and it was printed with a subtle logo from the Sundance Institute, a script-development workshop founded by Robert Redford that I was proud to have been a part of. Sundance was the last professional community I had bonded with deeply before becoming ill, and it was a major inspirational goal for me to return there as quickly as possible after I was well. Many of the friends who saw me through my treatments, who had called and encouraged me, I had met at Sundance. I commented silently to myself on the ridiculousness of branding colors with universal connotations. After all, my black sweatshirt was a reminder of some of my most treasured memories. How could it be harmful to wear something that made me feel good? I told myself that I was above those superstitions, that I had no need to play those kinds of games with myself and with my mind. And I didn't wear another stitch of black clothing for the next seven years.

The last few days at the Simonton Center were filled with even more good advice and solid techniques for, if not overcoming illness, at least managing it well. To Carl's credit, he noted this distinction and emphasized the equal importance of both. He imparted the familiar wisdom that just as important as long life was the courage to live fully the life one had left — and neither Carl nor any of his staff was ever at a loss for an aphorism to illustrate their points. "More perfect in being, than trying to be perfect." "The process of struggle needs to be worthwhile." "It's not what I do, but how I *think* about what I do." "Be committed to beliefs, but not attached." "The opposite of TRUST is FEAR." The collection scrawled on the meeting room's blackboard was truly impressive. Most of the slogans, in the context of the lectures, managed to avoid the patronizing quality of the platitudes they so closely resembled. They were enthusiastically, if less than judiciously, used as helpful illustrations of whatever concept was being discussed. But one of these trite sayings went far beyond the realm of illustration and became a source of illumination by itself. It made an instant impact on me and has remained a challenge to live up to ever since.

In the midst of a compelling talk about relationships, including an analysis of the concepts of "rescuing" others when help is not asked for, and thereby "victimizing" oneself when their gratitude is insufficient, one of the therapists made a pronouncement of an infallible technique for happiness in life and peace in personal relationships. His words took my breath away. Partly because he was right; it was a perfect formula. But on some intuitive level I must have also recognized the deceptive difficulty of this exquisitely complex equation.

"Always ask for what you want one hundred percent of the time. Be willing to hear no. Be willing to negotiate."

I wondered at the terror these three bland sentences threw into my heart. The simplicity of the message made it seem almost tender. But the design was hard-edged, and I knew instinctively that living up to the dare would be, unless I were to dramatically alter my ways, nearly impossible. I didn't know why always asking for what I wanted should be such an alarming proposition. It seemed to be a perfectly sensible way to behave. In fact, I couldn't quite pinpoint when, or why, I had stopped doing just that. I don't know what effect, if any, this tidbit from the week at the Simonton Center had on the other participants. But for me, it began to alter my life almost immediately. Especially in that great bastion of negotiation and compromise: the long-term romantic relationship.

Jackie and I were deeply in love. On page after page of the notebook I kept through the first six months of treatment, I had written about my love for her. In trying to outline graspable goals for myself beyond our time at the Simonton Center, I wrote about our future together. I spent hours visualizing images of domestic bliss, symbolizing the depth of our love. I imagined our children and held fatherhood out to myself as the ultimate purpose in life; the foremost reason to persevere in spite of anything that might happen. We would both fantasize, hour after hour, about parenthood. We laughed at each other for the ways in which we expected the other to be an overprotective mom or dad. We poked fun at each other's worst physical characteristics, blaming the other in advance for the agony our imagined offspring would have to endure in elementary school for having such a funny nose; such giant elephant ears. Jackie seemed proud of me for the way I had handled the catastrophe my life had become, and I was something much more than proud of her. I felt that I had been granted the privilege of sharing my time with the most generous, admirable, like-minded woman the world had to offer. A woman who, when times got tough, was capable of feats of strength I had only heard told in legends from the past. One of the dominant goals I had set in confronting the adversaries that consumed my recent past and my forseeable future was to forge an enduring love with Jackie — the love of my life. The only problem was, in the weeks leading up to and including our Simonton stay, we never had sex anymore.

Confronting death before I had gotten to form a secure sexual identity for myself had felt like one of the most frustrating and tragic aspects of the whole episode. Many of my pledges over the past six months had revolved around eliminating what now felt like the ridiculousness of the inhibitions surrounding my sexuality. Indeed, during months spent locked away from life, wondering whether I'd ever get another chance at it, any type of timidness or reluctance had come to seem like a ludicrous waste of opportunity. The reason for living was fantasy fulfillment, I concluded. I had made the mistake of tiptoeing my first time out, but I wouldn't play the fool twice in a row. I promised myself that if I got my time back, I was going to become the free, adventurous being that I'd always wanted to be.

This formed an important aspect of my earlier and ongoing therapy in New York with Dr. Patten, my "death therapist." In counseling me to deal with the issue of my own mortality and the possibility of its imminence, he also helped me explore the converse occurrence: How would I deal with life if I were able to get it back for myself?

My answer to that question was to launch into a laundry list of "never agains." Never again would I settle for apathy or discontent; no longer would I allow other people's fears to intimidate me; from now on, I swore, I would insist on boldness and candor not only from myself, but from anyone who wanted to spend time with me. I issued the challenge to myself in Dr. Patten's office to seize hold of life and wring every drop of drinkable moisture out of it. I was going to explode out of the starting block, and anyone who couldn't keep up would simply have to be left behind. Dr. Patten's response to my weekly harangue was a languorous, admiring half-smile, followed by another question.

"Well. You've certainly made it very risky for yourself to survive, haven't you, Evan?"

For a while, Jackie and I had kept a sex life going, even in the hospital. At first, when the shock of the diagnosis was fresh and our fear of losing each other caused a swelling in the intensity of our feelings, we fooled around on a pretty regular basis. The difficulty of accomplishing that was one more indignity that we latched onto as fuel for our outrage over the conditions of confinement. Hospital sex became a militant act. "We are young, vibrant people," we would rail on to each other. "How dare they deny us any privacy, any access to a space where we might feel comfortable to engage in what is probably the most life-affirming activity available to a human being?"

Since the powers that ruled the hospital had given no consideration whatsoever to creating an atmosphere in which pleasurable intimacy was easily accomplished, we decided that we would put into practice a similar system of carelessness. If nurses and doctors and technicians felt there was no imaginable reason to knock before entering a patient's room, then it wouldn't be our responsibility to shield them from what they might find inside. We were presumptuous enough to believe that we would be providing a valuable lesson to the staff. If they happened upon us in full coital combat, we reasoned, maybe they'd think twice next time before assuming that all their patients were nothing more than sexless vessels of disease. Unfortunately, the interruptions were so frequent — an uninterrupted series of interruptions, one could accurately say — that this crusade proved more frustrating than satisfying. While various unwelcome interlopers would routinely happen upon us snuggled into my hospital bed together, the amount of time between intrusions wasn't enough to achieve even a mild level of arousal. In the end, we did what, I suppose, was expected of us all along. We moved into the bathroom.

In we would lumber, I dragging my IV pole loaded with twenty pounds of liquid behind me, to begin groping our way toward some level of gratification. With Jackie's leg propped up on the toilet bowl, me clutching the cold metal support bar on the wall for leverage, we would triumphantly stake our claim to our right to consummate our love for each other. When things really got swinging in there, when we were both good and tangled in the tubes feeding me fluids, and banging our heads against the paper towel dispenser, one of us would inevitably knock against the little lever and the loud roar of the toilet flushing would send an extra little shiver up and down our spines.

It is remarkable, the extent to which one's surroundings can disappear when in the grip of sexual energy. Those were the only moments when I was able to even partially forget where I was and be fully engaged in the moment and activity at hand. Not surprisingly, however, there were times when bringing sex into the situation only added to the unreality of our existence. Either sitting on the toilet bowl myself, with Jackie leaning back into me for support, or standing behind her as she gripped the sink with both her hands; with the smell of powerful disinfectant burning my nose and the sounds of hospital business ringing in my ears, I would watch as the waves of orgasm tore through her. I wondered whether she was oblivious, in those few instants, to the circumstances that had led her toward those twelve seconds of bliss. It seemed incomprehensible to me that she could be feeling anything other than mortification over this arrangement.

I sometimes caught myself stumbling into sadomasochistic imaginings surrounding her inner turmoil. Much like one might prod a painful loose tooth with his tongue, I would convince myself that Jackie was pretending her pleasure and giving me the gift of her performance out of some misguided sense of pity. Then I'd become angry and, in the privacy of my mind, I would relish the opportunity to debase her in this way. Other times, I would just stare at her, marveling at the miracle of the woman. I would study her face, only inches from the drain as she stretched to squeeze the spasms out to every fiber of her being, and I would send myself out of that narrow cubicle and float off into space. Looking down from high above, I would no longer experience the building as a hospital, or the room as a bathroom. I would only see two small creatures, dwarfed by their surroundings to an extent unimaginable to them, busily engaged in a frantic activity that, seen from a distance, had no discernible significance at all. None, but for the desperate determination burned into their faces.

Eventually, blow jobs in the bathroom and tubes, illness, and frailty took their toll on Jackie. By the time I left the hospital after round three, she had become my caretaker and my partner, but lovemaking had been, for some time, an activity we shared only rarely. I was well aware of the old adage that says "When the patient recovers, the nurse falls ill," and it was fast becoming much more than a trite aphorism back at home with us. For the last three months or so, even during the periods when I was well and strong enough to enjoy sex, it had become a subject surrounded by tension and discomfort. What had at first presented itself as a series of painful attempts at intercourse was eventually diagnosed as a vaginal infection, and it stayed a vaginal infection. For weeks. For months. When we discovered that Jackie's "infection" had never really existed, and that the cause of her discomfort was actually a common allergic reaction to a contraceptive product, our problems were not alleviated by banishing the culprit. Jackie continued to be unwilling to attempt any sexual contact. If she could be coaxed into trying, she would lie rigidly beneath me, completely unresponsive, looking traumatized and on the verge of tears. Any attempt to talk with her about it, any inquiry into what might be bothering her, resulted in Jackie lapsing into a state of total silence and emotional paralysis.

My mind raced wildly over all the most unbearable possibilities. In the latter part of the last six months Jackie had been taking better care of herself by taking days and nights off every so often. I completely understood her need for some relief from her incessant caretaking. But I would still be seized by feelings of fear and inadequacy when male friends of Jackie's, and often my own good buddies, would arrive to take her away from me and the hospital to go out and have a good time. After they'd left me alone for the night, I would begin to construct the most painful explanations possible for our problems.

What if Jackie never had an infection at all? I wondered. Wasn't it possible that Jackie was hiding the fact that she had become pregnant over the past few months? I groomed and cared for this fantasy like a masochist's good luck charm. I embellished it, weaving in the detail of the abortion she'd had, and how she was keeping the whole thing from me to spare me any more grief than I was already suffering.

Once I had settled on this particular method to best torture myself, it was a breeze to pollute my thinking even further. I began building upon this scenario, deciding that Jackie had kept the pregnancy from me not to spare me conflict over the dilemma, but rather because she knew that I was not the one who had caused it. I would shuffle my plot lines daily, imagining first that one particular friend had seduced my girlfriend while I lay dying. The next day I might cast Jackie as the villain, playing explicit films in my head of her initiating a liaison with another of my closest comrades. Occasionally I would give myself a break, content to stop with the comparatively comfortable thought that the reason Jackie hadn't told me about her "pregnancy" and its termination was as benign as her desire — should I happen to survive the illness — to leave me as soon as I was well.

I suppose it might have been easy enough to slice through this swamp of morbid self-pity. After all, I could have just asked Jackie if any of these events had taken place. But I was bound up by a more complex collection of knots than ordinary jealousy. I was, I believe, involved in an intricate method of working through the extraordinary level of helplessness I was feeling. All my efforts at maintaining control of my situation fell far short of accomplishing any true independence. The fact was, by this time, I had come to rely on Jackie for the only pleasure I experienced. A better recipe for sexual problems would be hard to come up with.

My only power existed in the privacy of my own thoughts; hence, the retribution I sought in my angry assumptions of her nonexistent betrayals of me. Simultaneously, I was ashamed of the ways I was succumbing to the strain. So I kept my insecurity-driven suspicions to myself, concluding that if that's what she needed to get herself through the crisis; if that's the sustenance she needed in order to rescue me, who was I to complain? I didn't want to do or say anything that might drive her further away.

Walking the trails and pathways of Temescal Canyon; sitting through one Simonton workshop after another; and then each evening with Jackie back in our grungy bungalow, I was becoming increasingly exasperated with the status quo at work in our relationship. It wasn't so much the problems we faced that were unacceptable to me, but the silence surrounding them. Jackie seemed to have instituted a hard, unspoken rule against broaching the topic, and, whenever that rule was broken, she would disintegrate. I was left trying to reconcile the promises I had made to myself in my death therapy sessions and the "Always ask for what you want one hundred percent of the time" mantra with the meek acceptance I was practicing in the privacy of my life. During the long evenings spent alone together in our cabin, with nothing to do but talk — about the day, about our classmates, about ourselves and each other — I was covering every conceivable topic but the one that was on my mind. And, try as I might, I couldn't get Jackie to open up and begin a dialogue about what was bothering her. It wasn't that she was unwilling; that much was clear. She was simply unable. Any mention of the problem, any search for an opening for a discussion, resulted in her collapsing into a frozen silence. Jackie was petrified, and any attempt I made to encroach upon her well-defended psyche, no matter how gentle the approach, was responded to as if it were an overwhelming attack.

Had it been another time in my life, I might have simply waited to see where things might go. Had the events of the past six months not occurred, there is no telling how I might have reacted. But at that particular juncture in my existence, I was under the spell of the theories and slogans that had served me well so far. I might not be able to choose what happened around me, but I could decide how I would respond to it. Any failure on my part to live up to the beliefs that I'd latched on to, at this point, felt like a potential threat to my life. I decided that I was not going to forgo anything that might help me to maintain the remission I was in, and I stopped cooperating in the unspoken pact Jackie and I had made about the problems we were facing. While the risks were great, toward the end of our week at the Simonton Center, I turned the same uncompromising scrutiny that I'd brought to everything so far to Jackie, and to our life together back home. For the first time in our relationship, I started to complain.

At first, nothing else really changed. Nothing was transformed, and our evenings continued along their usual patterns. The only difference was that now, when Jackie started to cry, I didn't stop talking. I went on and on about what it was that I wanted from her; how important it was to me that we find happiness together; and how much I wanted to make love with her. I told her that I didn't understand what the problems were and that I would need her help in trying to solve them. I talked, and talked, and talked. And Jackie cried. Oh, how she cried. When she did speak, it was usually to say something along the lines of "I don't know."

"What's wrong?"

"I don't know."

"If you knew what was wrong, would you tell me?"

"I don't know."

"Why are you crying?"

"I'm upset."

"What are you upset about?"

"I don't know."

Believe it or not, this was some kind of improvement. And even as Jackie became more and more aggressive in her defensiveness, I tried to believe that this was an improvement as well. Eventually, as communication improved slightly, Jackie shared with me some of her fears. She told me she perceived each of my entreaties as a subtle threat. To Jackie's mind, inherent in my insistence upon opening up our problems to discussion was an ultimatum: either we find a way to address difficult issues or Evan will leave.

Our last few evenings at the Simonton Center were spent having chilling arguments like none we'd had before. Then we'd spend the next day smiling with the others, holding hands and laughing with the group. For the first time in my life I was walking through my days wondering at the bizarre disparity between a couple's private persona and their public facade — and the couple included me.

Our Temescal Canyon adventure ended, as promised, with a night-time fire walk. All the seminar participants gathered on the lawn of the Presbyterian Church Retreat, along with the staff members and some friends of the center that had been invited. There were what looked to be Native American drums and other musical instruments scattered about, and the ceremony started with a communal New Age jam session beside a crackling fire that sent sparks swirling around our heads. After some singing and drumming, during which most of the seminar participants looked somewhat pained and uncomfortable, we were gathered around the hot coals for our demonstration.

I had been extremely curious about this fire-walking business. All week it had been held out as the ultimate illustration of nearly every theory that was being passed along to us. The main tenet of Simonton's philosophy was simply that people could change their belief systems at will. If one could imagine something as a reality, Carl would say, then it is just one more step to creating it as such. Walking across burning hot coals without suffering injury certainly challenged everything I had accepted as factual in my life. And all week, at each reverential mention of the hallowed event, my thoughts were, Sure. I'll believe it when I see it.

And I *wanted* to believe it. Hell, I wanted to believe in every kind of magic and marvel that I had ever heard about. It would have given me a much greater sense of security than the tenuous one I was trying so hard to manufacture now. But I couldn't. It didn't come naturally to me. Maybe it was the result of having grown up so close to Manhattan. I was a native New Yorker, and in New York, skepticism is a necessary survival mechanism. I had already done a remarkable job of creating belief in all kinds of unprovable methodology — my healers; my visualizations; meditations; the Simonton Center itself — but each new addition required its own elaborate "prove it to me" test period. So I was excited about the fire walk. I wanted it to be something that would force me to reexamine my suspicious nature. But I was just as prepared to have a good laugh at a lame attempt at some kind of spiritual optical illusion.

"Cool moss. Cool moss. Cool moss."

Jack, one of the instructors, was cooing into the ear of a young, blond woman — our visiting fire walk specialist. She was standing, as we all were, barefoot in the cool, wet grass. I was stationed several feet back from the heat of the ember-filled trench, while our demonstrator was perched at the near edge of the rectangle. After a few minutes, the blond woman, her eyes closed, began chanting along with Jack. Their voices melded into a soothing mantra.

"Cool moss. Cool moss. Cool moss."

As Jackie and I giggled, with Jack holding one of the blond woman's elbows and Barbi, across the bed of coals, holding the other, they took off and walked her briskly, but deliberately, through the center of the length of the trench. Back on the grass at the other end, she quickly wiped her feet in the dewy green blades, to make sure no coals clung to them, and jumped up and down, shrieking with enthusiasm and exaltation.

"Oh! I wanna go again. I wanna go again," she said.

I stood rooted to my spot, my gaze fixed on the path she had walked. I ignored her celebration, and I stared at the trench filled with coals. I had watched them build the bonfire about ten feet away. I had watched them carry the hot coals in shovels from the base of that fire to fill the trench. I had been present for the entire time they waited for the coals to turn from bright red to gray, but by no means had they cooled down much. I could still feel their heat from several feet away, and whenever the wind blew, the coals still managed to glow a deep orange-red in response. My mind raced to supply acceptable explanations for what I'd seen. The first to rush into my head was that Jack and Barbi had carried the woman across. While posing simply as "spotters," they had actually supported her weight. But I had watched carefully, and I had seen the woman's feet sink into the coals with each step, causing an unmistakable imprint as the embers were pushed down and to the sides. I had watched her weight provoke the clouds of sparks that had wrapped themselves around her ankles. Then I thought about her feet.

"I bet the bottom of her feet are callused," I said to Jackie. "She does this all the time, and the bottoms of her feet are probably scorched into hard leather." And then I watched Jack walk through the coals. And then I watched Barbi. And then they turned to us.

"Anyone else want to try?" we were asked.

Are they crazy? I thought. This is the most irresponsible thing I've ever seen.

During the course of the week, the frailties of most of the seminar participants had become clear. While we might have been able to pull off the appearance of strength for an afternoon or so, over the length of our stay, most of the folks had fallen prey to some bout of not feeling terribly well. I couldn't believe that these people were being encouraged to attempt something that was so obviously dangerous. I also couldn't imagine who would take them up on their offer. When Donna, the wig woman, stepped forward, I was flabbergasted.

Donna had come to the center very shortly after having been treated for ovarian cancer. She was clearly the next youngest participant to me, although I would have guessed her to be about ten years older than I was. Donna had spent the week quietly, often appearing to be weak and, at times, complaining of nausea from her last chemotherapy treatment. She was the last person I would have expected to walk across a fifteen-foot bed of glowing hot coals.

But I understood her desire. In the desperate situations we all shared, we were searching for any advantage we could find. We had just spent a week convincing ourselves that expanding our beliefs would be to our benefit, and here was an opportunity to blow old belief systems apart with the force of an atom bomb. If we could control our bodies to the point where 850-degree coals didn't burn our flesh simply by imagining we were strolling through a patch of "cool moss . . . cool moss . . . cool moss," what could a few errant cells do to us? The opportunity to prove our dominance over the bodies that were betraying us was as tempting as if someone had offered a swallow of curing serum. As Donna lined herself up, nervous and giggling, I pushed my way right to the edge of the pit, wanting to inhale her triumph, should she make it to the other side.

Jack coached her in one ear, Barbi in the other. "Okay, Donna," Jack said. "Just close your eyes and imagine you're standing in a patch of cool moss. That's all you have to think about, what your feet are feeling."

Barbi picked up her cue. "Donna, just tell yourself that all you will feel for the next few minutes is cool moss under your feet. Say it with us now. Okay, Donna? Say it with us."

I stood watching the three of them. Donna had her eyes closed, and Jack and Barbi were feeding their voices into her ears like two birds regurgitating food into the beaks of their blind chicks. Then they all chanted together, "Cool moss. Cool moss. Cool moss."

Donna stood poised on the brink a bit longer than the previous walkers had, but eventually, much to my own amazement, she plunged in and forged ahead. She tromped her way through the coals and out the other side. This time, as she whooped and celebrated back in the grass, so did everyone else in the group. It was as if she had liberated the rest of us. Delivered us from having to accept the narrow "factual" realities of our predicaments. There was no reality any longer, no hard truths, no indisputable facts. When 850-degree coals don't burn human flesh, science ceases to be of significance. Nothing is indisputable, nothing is inevitable, and nothing, nothing, is impossible.

I left the Simonton Center on a terrific high of optimism, tempered with just a touch of chagrin. Watching Donna, and the few other seminar participants who had made their way across the coals, had swelled the capacity of my receptors to absorb thoughts and ideas I would have previously dismissed as ludicrous. I felt primed for exploration, determined to seek out more and more similarly mind-expanding experiences until, one day, the example of my life itself would serve as an improbable, though irrefutable, reality for others. My confidence in the existence of powers beyond those I was practiced in had grown tremendously during the week. But, even considering the value of that growth, I still had to contend with its limits, and the way that the expansion had ground to a halt.

Before dousing the hot coals with water and extinguishing the hope-spewing embers for the night, Barbi — who, after my initial skepticism, I'd come to appreciate more and more during the week — had tried to convince me to take a turn walking the fire myself. I was already so captured by the desire to do it that I was hopping up and down on the sidelines, screaming with each successful pass by someone else. But every time I considered moving over to the starting line, I couldn't stop thinking of all the logical consequences of the move. As I said, I had been sprung free from the hospital only about a week before coming to California. Every imagining of a step off the grass and into the scorched channel brought visions of blistered flesh; of bandages and ointments. Worst of all, it brought up the possibility of winding up back under the control of doctors and bureaucrats, stripped of all rights and individuality. No matter how much I wanted to believe what I was seeing; no matter how much I was able to believe what I saw happening to others; whenever I imagined myself stepping away from what I had always held as undeniable, I couldn't trust in anything else as much as what I had learned from the first twenty-four years of my life — that hot coals burn people. I had to wonder if an inability to believe that my mind could protect my feet from the fire in Temescal Canyon wouldn't affect my ability to escape the other one that was still burning all around me.

EYE OF THE HURRICANE

Just before leaving for the Simonton Center, I had made the decision to remove myself from the experimental protocol study at Sloan-Kettering. The protocol had called for half the patients to receive what was referred to as "maintenance" chemotherapy. This meant that, for a period of one year after completing the final course of intensive "consolidation" chemo, half the patients on the study would continue to receive weekly injections of low-level chemotherapy on an outpatient basis. Theoretically, these injections would not adversely affect the patient's ability to enjoy life, and might even offer the possibility of extending the length of what was expected to be a limited period of remission. However, as the treatment was being given experimentally in order to gather statistical results, the only guaranteed beneficiaries of my injections would be the state of medical knowledge and those individuals who followed after me.

Since none of my relatives had proven to be an exact genetic tissue type match to me, there had been no way to perform what was already recognized as the most promising treatment for my leukemia — a bone marrow transplant. There is about a 25 percent chance of any sibling being an exact match, and, had that been the case, a transplant would have been the recommended treatment as soon as the leukemia went into remission. The two "consolidation" courses of chemotherapy were routinely given in the absence of a matching relative. This was what was referred to as "conventional chemotherapy."

However, recently there had emerged some new, experimental versions of bone marrow transplants that were either already being performed or just becoming visible on the horizon. We had learned, through research done by my mother, that some medical centers — such as the Fred Hutchinson Cancer Center, in Seattle, and Johns Hopkins Hospital, in Baltimore — were doing what were called "autologous" bone marrow transplants, meaning, transplants using the patient's own bone marrow. Fred Hutchinson was investigating transplants using relatives who were not exact tissue type matches or using bone marrow from donors who were not related at all. My mother, who by now had fully regained her gift for aggressive activism, had been contacting centers all over the United States, cataloguing their responses, and asking them for recommendations. She had spoken with dozens of doctors, not only those associated with hospitals, but also those affiliated with alternative therapy centers. She organized the information onto three-by-five-inch index cards and handed me the stack. After leaving the Simonton Center, I planned to make a trip to Seattle as a way of following up. I wanted to meet with some of the pioneers of the treatments and hear directly from them what my options were and what their recommendations would be.

Jesselyn Melman, my new doctor in New York, knew of my plans to visit some other medical centers. Dr. Melman, as opposed to Leonard Zweig, had been willing to spend some time during our visits discussing what I had learned about leukemia and the various treatments available. Just before leaving for California, when I informed her that I was declining any further treatment, she wasn't overtly supportive of my decision, but neither was she unsympathetic to it. Months earlier, when I'd asked questions about the advisability of the second round of consolidation chemo, I'd gotten answers that acknowledged a lack of scientific evidence of benefit. But, unlike with my current inquiries, I was told then that the doctors *suspected* the treatment plan was advisable. Of course, the doctors couldn't speak with authority, much less make professional recommendations, based on incomplete results of an unfinished study. So these variations were the subtleties of response that offered clues into the doctors' knowledge of how the statistics of a particular study were shaping up. Had there been any inkling on Dr. Melman's part that I might have been endangering myself, I felt confident that her response would have been clearly pointed in that particular direction. I often felt as if Dr. Melman and I were speaking in code.

However, while Dr. Melman was somewhat helpful when it came to answering questions put to her directly, she was not terribly forthcoming with any information that was not explicitly requested. When I inquired about the Fred Hutchinson Center and its work with monoclonal antibodies; or when I tried to discuss a Johns Hopkins Hospital study that had been published in the *New England Journal of Medicine* demonstrating a striking level of success after performing more than one hundred autologous transplants on patients with acute myelogenous leukemia in second and third remissions, Dr. Melman only nodded her head politely and complimented me on the thoroughness of my research. Then she told me that at Sloan-Kettering they would soon be performing their first two such transplants, adding, like an executive loyal to her firm, "And with our transplants, Evan, we'll be offering radiation!"

A consultation at the Fred Hutchinson Cancer Center, in Seattle, Washington, is like spending a day at an all-inclusive holiday resort.

Jackie and I arrived on a Tuesday for our first of several scheduled appointments, this one with a social worker. We were told there would be a bit of a wait, and we were seated in a small, comfortable waiting room that was filled with children's drawings outlining the history of their own, or a family member's, illness. The space was quiet, except for the sounds of the birds chirping in the trees outside the window, and we were the only people in the room.

When we were welcomed into the social worker's office, we were given stacks of booklets and written materials. The woman we met with was round and open-faced, friendly and eager to help. She outlined for us the length of stay should a transplant be decided upon, and the philosophies behind the Fred Hutchinson type of care; namely, that the patient and family must be kept together as a cohesive unit even though their lives would be temporarily uprooted, and that the best way to approach these changes was to keep everyone a well informed participant from beginning to end. This last aspect of the Hutchinson way was startlingly displayed when we traveled through the building to our appointment with the doctor. Lining the halls of the medical floors were very large, full-color photographs of patients and facilities. Some of the pictures were standard long shots of smiling, slipper-clad, baseball-capped bald people. Most of the pictures, though, were graphic medical journal close-ups of what lay ahead for those enrolled in the program. There were several photos of the ulcerated lining of a mouth; there were shots of blistering skin lesions; there were photos of patients isolated in protective plastic bubbles, where they had to remain for the better part of two months while their immune systems recovered from the devastation of a bone marrow transplant. Many of the pictures were not easy to look at or easy to decipher quickly. The damaged flesh was so distorted that it took several minutes to puzzle out just what the photograph was showing. For this reason there were explanations posted describing the potential side effects displayed; the frequency of their occurrence; and, of course, the overall statistics for the procedures. This wall at the Fred Hutchinson Cancer Center most resembled a display in a museum commemorating the victims of war atrocities or of some particularly horrific industrial accident.

When the doctor at Fred Hutchinson, after hearing my history and assessing my plight, began discussing his knowledge of the research being conducted *all around the world*, I was taken aback. I had come to believe that, in the medical profession, such things simply weren't done. My experience as a patient so far had shown me that, while there might be a lot of information out there, access to it was limited and I would have to find my own way in. Even the *New England Journal of Medicine* itself is difficult to gain access to unless one is a doctor, and no doctor other than my psychiatrist had ever offered to find articles or research papers for me. The message, as I understood it, seemed to be "Yes, we want you to get well. But we don't want anyone but ourselves to get you there, or to get any of the credit for it." And so I was even more surprised when the doctor at Fred Hutchinson began talking about the Johns Hopkins study, comparing it favorably to the Hutchinson program for my particular problems, and ended the consultation by saying that, as far as he could tell, Johns Hopkins seemed like the place that could help me the most. His recommendation was that Jackie and I take one more trip on our fact-finding mission and visit with them there. When he openly complimented a "rival" institution by saying, "They seem to be doing what you need. And, hey, you can't do any better than them," I wondered if this was a generosity common to the Pacific Northwest or if this doctor happened to be of a particularly radical breed. We thanked this man with a profusion that had to puzzle him, and we packed up and headed to Baltimore.

Jackie and I visited Johns Hopkins when the hospital was beginning to perform autologous bone marrow transplants on patients in first remissions. Until that point, due to the riskiness of the procedure, transplants were performed only as a last resort on patients who had already relapsed and gained a second, or even a third, remission. I had come looking for information to help me decide if I should be one of the first to jump right into the transplant arena or take my chances with the 80 percent probability of a recurrence. At that time we met with a doctor named Rein Saral, who stunned us by graciously inviting us into his office at precisely the agreed-upon hour of our appointment. After all my experiences at Sloan-Kettering, after all the debasing episodes in their outpatient clinic, this was the first time that I had ever been seen by a doctor without enduring an excruciatingly long wait.

I sat down across a cluttered wooden desk from Dr. Saral and looked up to notice a small framed drawing hanging over the light switch on the wall. The drawing was a simple rendering of a hammer, poised at an angle suggesting an imminent blow. The hammer was labeled with the letters "BMT," and below it, at the bottom of the picture, was the printed message "When all you have is a hammer, everything looks like a nail."

I repeated the saying in my head a few times while I stared at the picture. Slowly, through my confusion, I recognized that the letters "BMT" stood for bone marrow transplant.

"Just a little reminder," Dr. Saral said. I hadn't known that he'd noticed me studying the drawing. "It helps keep us honest."

"When all you have is a hammer, everything looks like a nail." I was astonished. I was an in-the-flesh, first-person witness to a group of doctors, or, who cares? just one doctor, who framed and hung a cartoon for the purpose of reminding himself to question his own judgment! I almost laughed out loud right there in his office. I wanted to run around the desk and hug this man. I wanted to throw my arms around him and be held. I turned to Jackie on my left and found her staring back at me with her own expression of wonder. If the look on my face was anything like hers, it was screaming, Did you see what I just saw?

We then proceeded to have an unhurried meeting that lasted more than ninety minutes. Dr. Saral never made any attempts to do anything other than to help give us as much information as possible about all my options for future treatment. The meeting became an exchange of ideas, as the doctor began to recognize the level of knowledge that Jackie and I shared about leukemia. In fact, our knowledge seemed not only to impress this man but to inspire him to share more of his own expertise with us. It wasn't that he was any more encouraging than anyone else; he had only the same cold, hard facts at his disposal — basically, that my life was probably almost over. The difference was, those facts didn't seem to make him want to run away from me. Just the opposite. He seemed genuinely eager to help while openly recognizing that the amount of help available was limited. In addition, he was quick to acknowledge the difficulty of the decisions that we were confronting, and sympathetic to the strain that we were under.

After all the travel, after all the phone conversations and all the reading, it was a simple decision that landed in my lap. Was I prepared to immediately enter a new hospital for a procedure that might substantially increase my chances for a permanent cure but that carried at least a one-in-five chance of killing me before I ever got out again? Or, was I ready to dive back into life, with the full knowledge that 80 percent of those in my situation suffer a recurrence of the disease within a short period of time? I started to weigh the pros and cons of each choice.

If I went to Johns Hopkins and had the transplant right away, should I survive the procedure, I would then be in a group out of which about 50 percent would be expected to remain free from disease. That meant, with the 20 percent mortality risk of the transplant factored in, the procedure offered, from beginning to end, about a 40 percent chance of a cure. That seemed a large increase from 20 percent. In addition, the Hopkins study suggested that almost all recurrences happened within one year of the transplant.

In my present situation, the only way to know if I would turn out to be one of the lucky few who never relapse was to go on living and wait. After about five years or so, the graph shifts dramatically, and the chances of relapsing become minute. That seemed an awfully long time to endure Damocles' sword hovering over my head. On the other hand, it was a harsh proposition indeed to think of going into the hospital once again, quite possibly dying there, when I might already be in the group destined to remain well from the treatment I'd already had. I became obsessed with the numbers and the calculations as I tried to sort out my options. The mundanity of the statistics I was juggling all day, as opposed to the existential depth of their repercussions, made for one of the most surreal periods of my life. And it couldn't have been very easy for the people around me. A social inquiry as innocent as "How are you?," regardless of the company, would often lead to an intricate assessment of my stastistical calculations for my own chance of survival. When I'd finish my impromptu presentation, the entire group would sag into a stunned silence. I'd be mortified, silently vowing that in the future I'd keep my problems to myself. The next day, in front of a different group of friends, I'd repeat the scene all over again.

Meanwhile, I would become furious at myself for giving so much credence to statistics of what had happened in the past to people other than myself. I tried to keep in mind that my situation was unique, and that I had abilities that no equation could calculate. I wanted to make a decision based on my own potential and beliefs, not out of fear over what had happened to someone else. However I would do it, I had to make up my mind; not about what to wear, or where to live, or who to date, or what to say — but about which weapon to choose. I had to determine how I was going to try to stay alive, and in doing so, I discovered that dying is not the only part of life that is inevitably done alone.

In the end, quite simply, I went with my heart. I remained true to the work that I had put in so far; to the faith that I had nurtured and grown out of nearly nothing. I reminded myself that I had been in the top 5 or 10 percent of almost everything I had done in my life, and so, in forgoing any more treatment, I still had a 10 or 15 percentage-point cushion to feel comforted by. The act of making the decision based on faith, especially since I'd started out as a completely faithless being, only strengthened the faith I had gained. I was through with hospitals and medication, with studies and statistics and the anxiety that they instilled. I was going to walk away and live my life, to create the life that I had promised myself, and to reap the rewards of transcending fear and expunging it from my existence.

In spite of our difficulties, Jackie and I had decided, during the last hospitalization, that we both wanted to be married when I was well. We cried together, and we spoke on and on about the wonderful life ahead of us. But, as her strength and spirit — her sexuality and sense of adventure — continued its retreat from me, I found myself mourning the life I'd locked myself out of with my predictable hospital bed proposal. Had I avoided death, I wondered, only to spend the rest of my days in a sexless marriage with a depressed partner?

I'm sure the memory of seeing her lover reduced to such helplessness for so long contributed greatly to Jackie's inability to feel remotely sexual within our relationship. In addition to that, I was aware of how difficult it must have been to open up again, to reinvest her love, in a prospect whose future was so dubious. I was certainly capable of recognizing these dynamics at work in our relationship. I was aware that the danger existed that Jackie might give of herself, identifying herself with my struggle, until she had no separate self left. I may even have had an inkling that it was just such a loss of independent identity that had rendered Jackie incapable of sexual desire. But, while I hoped that the passage of time would heal most of the wounds, Jackie was not the only one who was acutely aware of the ticking time bomb that might or might not be set to go off inside me. Time was the one ingredient that I simply, and absolutely, could not afford to grant her. Regardless of the debt that I owed her; no matter how much I would have liked to have been her hero the way that she had been mine; no matter what promises had been made, I needed to live — right away — because, with the odds stacked against me like they were, it might very well be my last chance. If Jackie was unable to seize hold of life, right now; if Jackie had to recover from the trauma of all that we'd just been through, I wished her well. But, to my way of thinking at the time, Jackie had the privilege of expecting a safe, secure future for herself. She would recover. If I waited for her, my time might pass me by. When all my feeble, amateur attempts to rouse her failed, in an act of utter desperation, I threw myself into an affair with another woman. When Jackie confronted me with my betrayal of her, I broke off our engagement and our relationship.

I left Jackie sobbing at the kitchen table of our apartment, and I went off to make a movie in upstate New York. *Sweet Lorraine* was a film that I had been cast in before illness had struck and that had gotten delayed in order to raise more financial backing. It was the story of a small, family-run, kosher Catskills resort hotel. The director, a man named Steve Gomer, had grown up in the very hotel where we would be filming. It had been owned and run by the family of his second cousin, Jane, who later became his wife. I had been cast to play one of a number of young summer staff members, the backbone of the hotel, in this film about the people and the lives behind the scenes of an all but extinct way of life. When the production resumed, it coincided perfectly with my decision to end my treatment, and I was thrilled by the serendipity of it all. I took it as an omen that I had made the right choice after all, and that one minute aspect of life had stopped speeding ahead and was waiting for me to climb back on. As I waited in the hallway for the elevator, I heard Jackie's cries from the apartment where I'd left her grow louder and louder. Between the wrenched gasps, I could hear her whimpering: "I don't want this to be happening. . . . I don't want this to be happening." The same words that I had cried myself to sleep with night after night in the hospital for months and months on end.

If I could have physically torn myself in half, I would have. Listening to Jackie pleading out loud, to no one, in an empty apartment, nearly did the trick for me. Standing in the grimy hallway, staring at the floor, I was able to see only two options: go back and try to save Jackie or save myself.

Fuck the elevator. I ran down the stairs.

The lush dampness of summer in the Catskill Mountains was the perfect climate to plant the seeds for a new beginning. The adventure began with a cab ride up to Broadway and Sixty-eighth Street, where I was dropped onto the deserted sidewalk just after dawn. It was early in May, but the temperature had soared in the past few days, so I was dressed in cut-off denim shorts. The morning air still held a damp chill, but it was clearly temporary, destined to be burned off long before afternoon. A hot summer day passing itself off as another cold spring morning. The flashbacks to the days when my parents dropped me off for summer camp were strong and only got stronger as one, and then another, of the cast members straggled around a corner or flopped out of a taxi to wait for our ride to the country. We approached each other cautiously, with no way to be certain that we belonged to the same club, except for the fact that we were the only humans on the street so early, and that we were each dragging enormous trunks and duffel bags, stereo music boxes, and other identity-proclaiming accoutrements. We made hasty introductions, laughed about mutual friends and acquaintances, and piled ourselves into a van for the three-hour drive.

As we left the city and any concrete clues to our previous histories behind I was grabbed by the thought that I could simply invent a new one for myself and my unknowing companions. Nothing from the past would apply over the next six weeks, I naively thought. Crossing the George Washington Bridge and speeding up the Palisades Parkway, listening to the others tell tales of how they had arrived at this moment in their lives, I kept quiet in the front seat next to the driver. The questions and the banter being thrown around behind me felt oddly threatening to my imagined secret identity. The blandness of innocuous questions such as "What have you been up to lately?" now possessed the power to blow my cover completely. I hadn't invented a story for myself before leaving home; indeed, I hadn't even thought about withholding any information until we got into the tight quarters of the van. Only then did I recognize the quandary that would confront me over and over for the next six weeks.

Of course, I could just be open and honest with everyone. Let them all tell stories of their winter's employment; explain the pain and sorrow of their latest love; bitch about the indignities of the business we shared. When it was my turn, I'd just turn around in my seat, smile, and say, "Oh, you know. I got leukemia back in late September. Been in the hospital since then. Got out a few weeks ago. They say I'll almost certainly wind up back there before long. Then I'll be dead soon after that. So I'm just trying to have as much fun as I can until then!" But I expected that, if half of them didn't leap out of the speeding vehicle to escape, such a statement might cast a bit of a pall over the forced intimacy of our first moments together. And it's not that I necessarily *wanted* to tell them exactly where I'd been for the past seven months, but I couldn't think of anything else to say. It was as if my life was empty of any experience that I could relate other than my recent struggle to survive. Not only was I completely bankrupt of my ability to engage in any kind of small talk, but I was keeping close tabs on a nagging aggravation I was feeling about all of theirs. I was beginning to squirm with impatience and jealousy as I listened to those vibrant young souls

giggling over the latest of their meaningless triumphs and disappoint-
ments. I felt worlds away from them as I sat, only a car seat apart,
hurtling along the New York State Thruway toward my future. It
was a future that we would all, to a certain extent, share. But the
past that would inform my slice of it left me feeling set apart, as if
I was inhabiting an entirely different time zone from the rest of them.

Immediately after being offered the role, I had been contacted to
go for a medical checkup, as are all actors contracted to work for a
week or more in a film. Production costs on a film set can range
up to hundreds of thousands of dollars per day. Should an actor
become unable to complete a shoot once he's been on camera for
three weeks already, it could bankrupt the production company. An
insurance policy is therefore taken out on each actor, so that, in the
event one becomes ill, the company can get reimbursed for its costs,
recast, and reshoot. When I was contacted about the physical, I
panicked. No insurance company would have covered me at that
point, just weeks after completing treatment, only seven months
after being diagnosed with an almost always fatal disease.

Steve Gomer's wife, Jane, worked as a physical therapist at Sloan-
Kettering. We had never met before, but I assumed she had something to do with easing her husband's concerns, and I was hired for
the job without a physical being required. Steve and his partners
were willing to take a chance on me, bringing me on board with no
insurance coverage, risking their entire production. This was a decision so far out of the ordinary it was difficult to imagine they knew
what they were doing. I was living life as a tightrope walk without
a net, but only because I had no other choice. The generosity of
Steve and the other producers, in their willingness to take that walk
with me, all so they could have me in their film, made the stakes
that much higher. I wanted to prove to Steve, and to the rest of the
world, that they had done the right thing. Whenever I worried about
my health over that six-week shoot, I was aware of the fact that I
was carrying a responsibility not only to myself, but to others as

well. Each night I would go to sleep and pray that I would make it through the schedule. I would count the days gone by like money safely in the bank, looking ahead to the shrinking number still to pass.

The first week in the Catskills was devoted to rehearsals and training. Each morning we would get up at the crack of dawn, change into our waiter's uniforms, and be driven over to The Pines, one of the fading Borscht Belt resorts. There we would trail one of the waiters or waitresses, trying to learn the techniques behind lifting forty-pound, food-laden trays with only the thumb and two fingers of one hand. Afternoons were spent reading and rereading the script, joking endlessly with each other, and tailoring our lines and roles to best suit our own particular sense of humor. It was Steve's idea, and his strength as a director, to give us wide leeway in our performances. As long as it made Steve laugh, we could do or say just about anything we wanted on camera.

The freedom of this atmosphere allowed me to relax right away. After the van ride up from the city, I decided that I wasn't going to allow anything to shut me out of this experience. Whatever gap needed to be bridged to find my way back to the childlike exuberance I saw around me, I was determined to cross it and keep on running when I hit the other side. And, most surprising of all, I was able to do it. I watched myself in amazement as I attacked everything put in front of me with a ferocity of spirit. I was overjoyed to find that, in spite of the isolation my experiences inflicted upon me, I was able to approach life in a much less inhibited fashion. The training sessions, the rehearsals, and the hours we all spent laughing and joking with each other were all imbued with a newness for me that resulted in my catapulting myself into them. I latched onto a Salvadoran waiter at The Pines who, like the character I was to play, was a freewheeling, fast-talking, horse-betting hustler. I watched as he good-naturedly charmed the elderly guests of the hotel and not so good-naturedly poked fun at them behind their backs.

"Decaf," he'd scoff, as he came back from a table and rushed over to the coffee station. "I'll give them decaf." Then he'd cut the full-strength, caffeinated coffee with 50 percent hot water and head on back to the table with a big smile for everyone.

His name was Henry, and I was awed by his ability to pick winning horses at the track. Then I'd laugh with him after he drunkenly misplaced the two hundred dollars I'd watched him win ten minutes before. I tried to adopt his reckless attitude toward life. He seemed to know that all that really mattered was the feeling of the moment, and he was a master at finding his fun there. For the first time in my life I was able to muster a little bit of the same skill. In my sly asides to loosen up the other actors between takes; in our all-out basketball games played on our lunch breaks; in my insistence on trying something different and new each time the cameras rolled, I was playing every moment out for all the juice that could be squeezed out of it. Dreaming about the future, however, which reminded me of its uncertainty, was something I could not allow myself to indulge in. And so I leapt at each moment as it was presented to me. It was the life of a man possessed.

Although I was having fun, laughing my head off a good part of every day, I felt as if there was no one there who really knew me. And I felt that they never would know me, unless I was able to tell them the truth about what had happened to me. When, in the midst of just one more van ride to or from a location, I happened to mention that I had spent most of the previous year in and out of the hospital, all heads swung in my direction.

"Why were you in the hospital?" someone asked.

"I had leukemia," I answered.

After a stunned pause, the questions began. I was surprised to find that rather than being repulsed by my history, people were intensely curious. Revealing the hidden details of my life didn't cause people to treat me as someone more delicate than themselves. Instead, I found myself being regarded with admiration. While I might have felt uncomfortable had they been respecting me only for having been ill, that didn't seem to be the case. At first I barely listened as one of my comrades said, "Wow, that's brave." It was an empty statement to me by this point, no more incisive or heartfelt than someone saying "Have a nice day." But when I heard her go on, I was moved. "Telling us about that the way you did," caught my ear as a fresh twist. "Just saying 'Hey, this is me' flat out like that. That is really brave."

It was my first taste of a new power, a new path, that wouldn't become clear to me for some time. My new friends were looking at me with a surprised esteem for having openly revealed to them the crux of my existence.

Just past midnight on July 1, after finishing a somewhat tedious sequence of shots, the assistant director of *Sweet Lorraine* called out, "That's a wrap!" and the filming was complete. I wandered out, in a bit of a daze, to the back lawns of the hotel where we had spent the last six weeks making the film. As I heard the cast and crew scrambling to finish their work so the party could begin, as the music wafted toward me from the ballroom of the hotel, I drifted farther and farther away from the sounds. My eyes were drawn up to the night sky, which was splattered with sparkling lights. The Milky Way was a solid, misty stripe cutting a swath across the darker background, where the lonelier stars throbbed their light toward me and my self-obsessed insignificance. I climbed on top of a picnic table and took off my shoes and my sweaty shirt. It had been broiling hot inside, under the film lights, but here in the cold mountain air, with only those distant fires burning in the sky, the temperature had dropped surprisingly low.

Standing on the picnic table shortly after midnight on the first of July, listening to the shouts of joy wafting their way out to me and hearing the corks popping on the champagne bottles, I had a celebration of my own. I stood, half-naked in the cold, and I screamed out into the night. I yelped and I howled at the stars and the moon, with a sense of joy and relief and accomplishment big enough to fill the sky above me. I had my celebration separately from the others because I had different things to celebrate. I hadn't realized, until the job was done, how frightened I'd been. That I might be interrupted. That my health might fail and ruin everything. But I had done it. This time the task begun had been completed, and it gave me a feeling that I'd never had so intensely before. I licked the salt from the tears that were rolling down my face and, out of breath and exhausted, I headed up the sloping grass to join the others, ready to take my place as one of them.

My separation from Jackie didn't last long. Neither did any of the others that we tried over the next several months. Jackie and I had come to equate our survival with our attachment to each other. Like an old couple who emerge from hiding after a long siege, Jackie and I both feared that it was the act of clinging to one another that had spared our lives. Never mind the fact that we didn't know how to live *with* each other. Letting go, even for a moment, made us feel exposed and vulnerable to the flying bullets and exploding bombs that we had dodged together so far.

We traveled to Europe. I made another movie. I had my triumphant return to Sundance Institute, where I was welcomed by the people I'd met just before falling ill. I lived loud and embraced my mistakes, and for the first time I felt great about all of it. Every aspect of life had become a terrific adventure. Something to be done, just to see what would happen. Even going to the dentist became a great way to spend the day, because it was part of life, and life was what I had wanted, and now it was mine. I'd sit in the dentist's chair, determined to *feel* everything. Enjoying the fact that I was there, privileged enough to have that needle piercing my gums. Feeling lucky to be smelling my teeth burning up under the drill.

This supercharged curiosity about life completely changed the way people responded to me. I would never have described myself as having a "magnetic personality," but the freedom I felt as a result of unshackling myself from the accepted constraints of behavior drew people toward me in ways and numbers I had never before experienced. As I breezed through my days indulging my whims, arriving places according to my own personal schedule, and speaking my mind with the candor of someone who had nothing to lose, I found myself surrounded by admirers who wanted to play along. I revisited the summer theater retreat in Tannersville where Jackie and I had met and, with no responsibilities to live up to myself, I encouraged others to abandon theirs. I was the "hooky mascot" that summer, available to sneak off with whoever might be ready to desert his or her post on any given day.

This dynamic crystalized a theory I'd held for a long time already: people are attracted to those who can afford to behave in ways they can't get away with themselves. It's a trait that runs through many of our celebrities, both in the characters they portray and in their own personal lives. Those who can brawl and sleep around, mouth off and back it up with heavy firepower allow the rest of us to vicariously experience the freedom that would leave us jobless and friendless if we ever truly embraced it.

And that's exactly what started to happen to me. The role that I had chosen to play in the immediate aftermath of my struggle, that of the "professional distractor," eventually set me apart from the same people whom I had lured in with it. Using the money I'd saved from *Sweet Lorraine*, I absolved myself from all obligations other than to myself. Traveling back and forth between Tannersville, New York City, Utah, and South Carolina — visiting friends, driving aimlessly for hours — I granted myself a respite from the pressures of time. I was free not only for the one afternoon I might have convinced one person to run off with me, but for every day afterward

as well. This laid the ground for resentment toward me when each
of my new friends went back to work and I continued to frolic. If
any intimacy had developed between us in our afternoon of abandon,
either romantic or not, there was the specter of jealousy as I repeated
my daily ritual with someone else the next day. If I did get myself
into an interpersonal scrape that felt too tempestuous for my mood,
I might just skip town the next day. The people I met during those
days seemed to be drawn in and repulsed in equal measure.

And there was still, of course, Jackie, who, after all the time she
had been forced to live without stability in her life, was probably
after anything but adventure in this phase of it. One by one, the
same people who had run after me either drifted away or expressed
the limits of their tolerance, for the very same reasons they had
sought me out to begin with. It started to become clear that I would
have a choice to make eventually between accepting the different
attitudes and priorities my experiences had instilled in me, and so
leading a life set apart from most others, and finding my way back
to the lives being lived by most of the people I cared about, and
assenting to the terms of the social contract most people tacitly agree
to without such conscious deliberation.

*   *   *

I had wondered, since the first day of the ordeal, whether the fact
that I'd been ill would affect my career. Would people less generous
and enlightened than Steve Gomer be reluctant to hire me, since I
had left a Broadway production because of illness? About a year into
my brand-new life, I got a call to go audition for another Neil Simon
play. If I could get back on Broadway, I thought, working for the
same people that I worked for before I got robbed, I'd be able to
feel like I had really reclaimed all the possessions of my life.

Down in the basement of the theater, I was sitting on the dirty
concrete floor with about six other actors. I had already read a couple
of scenes for Neil and Manny Azenberg and Gene Saks, the power
trio, and they'd sent me downstairs to look over another one. A

shadow blocked the light, and I looked up to see Manny, the producer, towering over me.

He said, "You're a breath away. Don't blow it."

I squinted up at Manny, and opened my mouth. Before I could make a sound, he said, "Don't blow it." And he walked away, back up the stairs.

I decided to take this as encouragement. I mean, it seemed like Manny was really rooting for me — in his own way.

And by the time I got home that day, I had the part. I went to the window and I screamed out into the sweaty New York air. I couldn't stop screaming. I don't think I had ever gotten as excited before in my life. Not in any way that I showed it. But I had gotten everything back, and more. I had fooled the angel of death and won back all my toys; all the possessions and freedoms that somehow added up and equaled my life. I had them all, once again, plus a brand-new spirit to enjoy them with. Everything felt complete, and for the next four months I basked in the luxury of my victory.

Perhaps "basked" gives me a bit more credit than I deserve. I was flying high with my newly reacquired Broadway swell status, and I wasn't shy about combining my victory proclamation with a cry of triumph over my health. "STILL ALIVE AND WELL: Evan Handler is back on Broadway in Neil Simon's *Broadway Bound*" read the ad I took out in the trade papers to announce my return. Each evening, at seven P.M. or so, as I rounded the corner of Broadway and Forty-fourth Street, I never failed to get misty-eyed and tingly when I saw the sparkling marquis of the theaters and passed through the stage door of the one I was appearing in. But, as far as keeping a fresh appreciation of life and its gifts, my attitude began to spoil quickly. In fact, as the boundless expectations I'd carried through my life once again took hold, it was swiftly turning rancid.

One of the most dependable follow-ups to landing any coveted acting job is the grim process of negotiating a contract. In one instant, the potential employer who has selected you after careful examination of every available alternative turns from your smiling admirer into your snarling adversary. After paying you the highest compliment possible, that of desiring your services, the employer begins to methodically catalogue all the reasons why your services are not worth very much. Business is business, and every negotiation I have been involved in has come down to the same extremely simple decision: Take it or leave it. And, if you can't afford to walk away and lose the job, you ain't gonna get what you think you deserve.

When I began my tenure in the cast of *Broadway Bound*, my disappointment over the fact that my salary was half that of my predecessor in the role was somewhat tempered by my inheritance of his dressing room. I am, unfortunately, an individual over whom the craving for status has influence to rival that of my desire to lead a life of thoughtful fulfillment. I hadn't been able to secure the salary I wanted for the job, my demands for equal billing to the actor I had replaced were laughed at, and the length of my commitment to the show was firmly imposed upon me. But, when I saw the palatial, luxurious dressing room I was being granted occupancy of — about the size of a small studio apartment, complete with sofa and easy chair and a modern bathroom with shower; when I saw that the room had both the space and impressiveness to function as a private, rent-free midtown office for the duration of the run, I was enthralled by the possibilities, and anxious to impress my post-show visitors.

Also in the cast of *Broadway Bound* was an older actor, an avid Socialist and political activist named John Randolph. John's career had already spanned several decades, despite a fifteen-year run on the Hollywood studio's blacklist of "subversives" in the 1950s and early '60s, and included appearances in dozens of major films through almost as many different eras. John's wife had died suddenly the year before, and John himself had recently undergone heart bypass surgery. In fact, he had begun rehearsals for the show only about two months after his operation. In spite of those hardships, John, for as long as I have known him, has been a man with the spirit and energy of a gleeful, if somewhat irascible, youngster. Both he and Linda Lavin had won Tony Awards for their roles in *Broadway Bound*, and John, upon accepting his award, had wished everyone watching on national television "Peace, love, and brown rice." Since the two of them had already been with the show for some time, they were both scheduled to leave the production after the first two months of my run. I was asked, in deference to his stature as one of our greatest actors, if I might be willing to let John use the stage-side dressing room until he left the show. Climbing the stairs to his room on the second floor was becoming a strain for him.

Of course, I didn't hesitate to say yes. It would have been ludicrous for me to think that, after a career such as John's, I was entitled to any privilege over him, regardless of the size of our roles in that particular play. And John was a great guy. He was constantly poking his head into my room and saying, "Tell me, son, are you interested in politics?" It didn't matter at all what I said back. The pamphlets were out in a flash, the latest news clipping was being analyzed, and John was picking apart someone's latest speech. If I was interested in politics, John was feeding my curiosity; if I wasn't, then it was his responsibility to educate me. Every now and again he would pause from his diatribe and look up with a smile as sweet as any child's.

"I know I'm boring you, but this will only take another few minutes. You're being very patient with me, I thank you."

With those two sentences he both sincerely apologized for his inability to contain his obsessions and cunningly mocked my complacency about the issues affecting my life. John Randolph was one of the most incredible characters I'd ever met. Walking down Forty-fourth Street toward Broadway with him was like strolling an electoral district with a born politician.

"Hello! John Randolph, the actor," he'd bellow, as he grabbed and shook the hand of anyone who might have vaguely made eye contact. John Randolph didn't worry about whether he was famous enough or not. He *assumed* everyone knew who he was, and that they were all eager to meet him.

So, while I was happy to give up my one contractual perk to Mr. Randolph, I was ashamed to discover how intensely the sacrifice affected my enjoyment of the job. Never mind that I was starring in a hit play on Broadway. Forget the fact that many of those in the audience each night were well aware of the remarkable journey I'd made to get back on the stage. And ignore the overpowering impression made on old friends when they traveled to the theater night after night, passing the dazzling lights and glittering names outside one theater after another. None of this mattered to me. I was depressed and frustrated by the fact that, for the first two months of my run, no one who stopped backstage to greet me would see me in the glorious surroundings in which they might have. My discontent was akin to that of a silly prince who, although everyone knows he is a prince and treats him like one, can't stop sulking on the days when his royal robes are out being cleaned. Apparently it wasn't enough for me to get to *be* on Broadway in a wonderful play. I needed everyone to see me wearing the Broadway suit of armor in order to feel that my shortcomings were well enough hidden away. I was aware of the grotesqueness of the ingratitude I was guilty of, and yet it seemed out of my control.

Once I had inherited the grand dressing room some weeks into my run, I learned that such irritations are rarely about the objects we project them on. I continued to find fault with one thing after another while I performed that play. It's not that I complained or made a nuisance of myself to anyone else, I just ruined my own experience. The safer I felt about my life and health, the more I demanded from the world around me, and within a very short amount of time, there was, once again, little that could please me.

Around this time, on a hot autumn day between appointments, I had a meal with my friend Ethan. This was a day on which I was spinning out of control. Furious. Fed up, once again, with the world and the friction that it inevitably inflicts on us. Ethan reminded me of another meal that we had shared, some months before, between hospital admissions. On that day, according to my friend, I'd said, "Ethan, if I ever get through this, I'm never gonna worry again. I'm never gonna worry, and I'll never hurry anywhere, ever again. I'm just gonna sit someplace green and watch the sun go up and down."

My friend Ethan reminded me of that, and all I wanted to do was punch him in the face as hard as I could.

I hardly got a chance to assess my friend Ethan's observation or my response to it. Almost two years to the day after the first diagnosis, I was found to have leukemia again. There were no beds immediately available in the hospital, so I kept performing in *Broadway Bound* for about another week and gave my last performance on Halloween. Jackie and I had a party to go to later that night and, in an attempt to imitate normalcy and nonchalance even greater than that shown by my going out onstage each evening, I went to the theater dressed as a rabbit. I was still wearing my bunny nose and my top hat with giant rabbit ears attached on the subway after the show, when a drunk man stopped in the aisle in front of us.

It's a terrible cliché, I know, but I've had a number of experiences in which filthy, red-eyed, drunk prophets have given me profound messages. Messages that seemed as if they couldn't have been meant for anyone but me. This man on the train stared at us, bleary-eyed, as he swayed back and forth. One hand held the handrail, as his other hand reached out and stroked the long, white ears that were growing out of my hat. The man's cracked lips twitched and grimaced as he studied me. Then he screamed:

"Were you exposed to nuclear radiation? You look like a genetic mutation. You know that? You look like a genetic mutation!"

CRYING JOB'S TEARS

Back inside Sloan-Kettering, I climbed into my bed in the corner room at the end of the hall and isolated myself from everything outside it. I accepted the fact that this time through, the treatment would be much more painful because I had no intention of investing in any positive attitudes again. Since the length of the remission had been twice the average, I had allowed myself to believe that there would be no more troubles. I had regained some of Jackie's trust in the last year, partly by not keeling over and dying on her; I had gotten the Neil Simon industry to trust me with the lead in his latest play; and I had just begun to trust the world again, myself. When my worst fears for my future became my reality, I found that I couldn't even allow myself the small measure of faith I had gained in my previous battles.

As far as I was concerned, I had suffered the very worst of the downsides of the self-actualization/healing philosophies. I'd allowed myself to believe I had the power to change the personality that inhabited the body that had bred the disease. I had believed that by "heeding the warning" of a drastic illness, I would be ensuring my safety in the future. I'd made changes; I'd learned to open myself more to love; I'd made great strides toward learning how to live. Why had I been stricken again? Already angry about the sense of failure I felt, I became even more enraged by the alternative "gurus" I had followed when I heard their denials that this was a real risk in the programs they outlined.

I saw Bernie Siegel and Louise Hay questioned together on an afternoon talk show, and I heard them state their beliefs that people were stricken with and died from diseases when they lost the ability to love themselves, or to feel and experience love in their lives. A young woman called into the show, and, shyly but with determination, she tearfully appealed to them for some understanding about the death of her brother.

"My brother died six months ago of leukemia, and before he died I bought him Dr. Siegel's book, and he really loved it; it was great and he kept thinking positive. He thought he was going to be okay. He had all the love in the world from the family, from all his friends, all the support. He had everything going for him. He knew what he wanted from life but he didn't make it and he never finished the book. So I want to know, why doesn't it work for everybody?"

It made me cringe to hear this woman begging a stranger to recognize her brother's love and knowledge of his own worth. Regardless of whether there was a point to be made or whether Bernie Siegel and Louise Hay have valid and important messages for patients — and I believe, to a large extent, that they do — I wanted so badly to see Dr. Siegel address the issue the woman had raised: that the statements he has made can and do make people feel that they may have failed somehow. Failed to feel and express love themselves, or failed to recognize the deprivation in those they care about. To my mind, no more proof was needed that this danger existed than the woman on the phone. If she felt the need to defend the level of love in her family, then something he said must have made her feel threatened. It may not have been his *intention* to do so, but I certainly expected to see him acknowledge that he had.

And the solution seemed so simple to me. I watched the pixels on the television screen as they imitated the image of the doctor, and I wished I could have whispered into his ear. I wanted to say, "Tell her people get tired. Sometimes people work as hard as they possibly can, and they learn lots of lessons and find a great deal of peace and happiness, yet, eventually, they get so tired that they just need to take a rest. And when you're sick, taking that rest can mean the end of life, as it will for all of us eventually." I know that when I thought I could no longer continue to fight, that was the reason.

Instead, Dr. Siegel simply stated, "The only thing that works for everybody is love. Then a part of her brother stays alive . . . if she has loved her brother, she has done what she can and now she has to go on." In all fairness to him I should say that I have heard Bernie Siegel state that none of his techniques or beliefs should be used to impart blame or promote guilt, and I believe he spoke the words at some point on that program. But I knew, as I watched that day, that many people *would* interpret his words that way, regardless of his disclaimer. And I knew that many would have devastating feelings of failure without any conscious interpretation at all. I knew that people would, in many cases, be left to wrestle with those feelings, by the author's intent or not — because I had become one of them.

Yes, I would endure much more pain this time around, I decided. But it would be the pain of a painful experience, lived honestly, without the narcotizing comfort of emotional sleight of hand. Now, those who came to visit me — those who were allowed admittance — were met by a mass of bitter, vengeful energy. I no longer made any effort to comfort the uninitiated, and if anyone tried to cheer me up, to brighten my mood, I mocked them mercilessly. I challenged them to defend the most inane polite chatter, daring them to come up with just one way things "could be worse," or to explain exactly why it was "good to see me." I spoke out loud my violent fantasies, pledging my future to a boxing career, openly relishing the thought of pummeling future opponents. I described in gory detail the bloody punishment I intended to inflict upon anyone unfortunate enough to come up against me. I was aware of the absurdity of these diatribes, coming from someone known to be, if not gentle, at least nonviolent — and weighing in at just over the weight of a moderately sized dog. So there was a kind of humor in my attacks. But it was always a testing humor, testing the limits of what the intruders could take. If they couldn't handle the depths of darkness to which my acrid asides would plunge, then I would become disgusted, and end the visit and the friendship in the same dismissive puff of breath.

I started to pride myself on this new outlook. I drew strength from my anger, deciding that it was now my mission to survive as a testimonial against all the comforting theories that had let me down. "Imagine," I would tell Jackie. "Imagine surviving leukemia with no faith in anything at all. An open admission that the world is a cruel, random place, where nothing matters beyond luck and ruthlessness." Those were the rock-hard thoughts out of which I carved my new will to live.

My new roommate was a young man named, if you can believe it, Willie Dingle. The first time I heard it, I thought, as far as his grade school existence must have gone, his parents might as well have named him Penis Penis.

Willie was somewhere close to my age, and he was a nice, friendly guy — but he was not doing well at all. He'd already had a bone marrow transplant, the procedure I was working my way toward, but Willie was not recovering properly. He was suffering from just about every complication one could hope to avoid, short of actually up and dying. Willie's hands and arms were wrapped in loose bandages, covering the sore, swollen tracks left by the endless attempts to locate his scarred veins, and he was constantly receiving some kind of blood transfusion. No matter how many platelets they pumped into poor Willie Dingle, his blood counts remained the same; no matter how many units of packed red cells they slipped under his skin, his body just burned them up without making use of them. As a result, one or the other of Willie's eyes was always stained an ugly bloody red from a burst blood vessel. As soon as one eye would heal, the other would spring a leak. With the bandages on his arms, his weary, plodding walk, and blood running out of his eyes, Willie looked like a full-color version of one of the zombies from *Night of the Living Dead.*

As a precautionary measure, the nursing staff had consigned Willie to strict bed rest. The platelet problem put him in extreme danger of hemorrhaging from the slightest bump or bruise. Regardless of the facts, every day Willie would get up to go for a walk, and quickly be led back to his bed by a gently scolding, soft-voiced nurse's aide.

"Now you know you not supposed to be out of bed, Willie. If you fall down or bump yourself, they ain't not one thing we gonna to be able to do for you."

It never stopped Willie, though. If he couldn't walk the halls, he'd wander around the room. I'd watch Willie round the corner of my curtain, making his way toward the bathroom we shared. He would lean heavily on his IV pole for support, sometimes stopping mysteriously to rest, or just to stand and think, somewhere along the eleven-step expedition. Whenever Willie parked himself near the foot of my bed, or stood staring wistfully out the window in the dead center of my line of sight, the silence in the room grew too real to tolerate.

"Hey, Willie," I'd say, just to be saying something. "How's it goin'?"

Willie would snap out of his trance, always looking surprised to remember where he was and that there was someone else there with him. Then he'd slowly drawl, his tired voice still stuck in whatever faraway place the rest of him had just returned from, "Ohhhhhh . . . you know," and he'd start back on his way, refreshed for the final leg of his journey across the barren desert of our semiprivate (whatever that means) hospital room.

That was pretty much the extent of our communication, Willie and I. Day after day, and sometimes several times within one:

"Hey, Willie. How's it goin'?"

"Ohhhhhh . . . you know."

Not that there wasn't variation within the form. Even without any other words than those, there is a respect and an intimacy that develops between people sharing in each other's illness and experiencing the looming possibility of each other's death. Willie and I never exchanged stories, we never gave each other a rundown of our personal histories. We never complained to, or relied on, each other. We overheard, and we witnessed, all of the very worst things that could possibly be happening to the other one. And once or twice a day I would say, "Hey, Willie. How's it goin'?"

And Willie would say, "Ohhhhhh . . . you know."

The doctors made their bedside visits at the crack of dawn. In the spooky illumination just beginning to seep through the window, the clomp of three pairs of shoes would penetrate my sleep just before the lights would snap on. The timing of the visits, I'm sure, was decided on for reasons no more malicious than efficient scheduling. But I couldn't help suspecting that, on some level, the doctors were glad to visit the patients when they were still asleep; the better to find them docile and undemanding, the better to drop their bombshells and make a quick getaway.

Early one morning, before the sun had even begun to rise, Willie was visited by one young female doctor, traveling alone. She padded around my bed, pulling the curtain to make an even tighter enclosure to seal me off from the other half of the room. She spoke to Willie without turning on the light. The doctor's voice was as hard and sharp as the floor tile in the predawn room. Her heavy suburban New Jersey accent was knocked off-kilter by an insistently sing-song perkiness and cheerful overenunciation she tried to inject into every sentence. The attempt was unfortunate. Instead of making her seem friendly, she only sounded bored. Instead of compensating for a lack of intelligence on her patient's part, she only called into question her own.

"Good mawning, Mistuh Dingle, how are you today?"

That question always got me. I never knew how to answer it myself, at five A.M., after being woken from a drug-induced sleep that I might have fallen into only a few hours before.

The doctor plowed on. "Mistuh Dingle, I'm Donna. Doctuh Gee's new fellow. We met yestuhday, remembuh?"

"Hnnn?" I heard Willie whine. I didn't think he was even awake.

"Mistuh Dingle, remembuh the CAT scan we took yestuhday?"

"Hnnn???" Willie's whine had tightened into a pleading whimper. It was the sound of someone fighting to stay hidden under the covers on a frigid morning, safe from the cold, and safe in sleep from life and its infinite indignities.

"The pictures, Mistuh Dingle, with the machine, of yuh head? Remembuh the pictures we took, Mistuh Dingle, of yuh head?"

"Hnn-nnnn . . ." I heard Willie make the sound again, but this time it was a surrender. A reluctant acceptance of the inevitability of whatever might be waiting for him.

"Well, Mistuh Dingle, there was a mass, okay? The pictures showed you have a mass. So we can't give you any more treatment until we find out what it is, okay? Mistuh Dingle? The pictures showed you have a mass." The way she said the word "mass" made me dig into my mattress with my fingernails. She honked the word out, with a harsh, compressed nasality that threatened to shatter the window panes and lightbulbs in the room. I heard Willie move in his bed. I couldn't tell if he was sitting up to pay more attention or pulling the pillow over his head, trying to pretend this woman was just a monster in some bad dream.

"Mistuh Dingle, I have a form here for you to sign. Since you have a mass, Mistuh Dingle, I need you to sign this form for us. Do you unduhstand? The form tells us what to do if you become incapacitated, okay? Do you unduhstand? Mistuh Dingle? The form tells us what to do if you become incapacitated. The form tells us if you want us to take extraordinary measures to resuscitate you, if you become incapacitated."

The word "incapacitated" had lost all its meaning for me. She said it so many times, in such a brief span, that it had become nothing more than a chunk of six-syllable gibberish. I assumed that Willie was at least nodding his head, because then the doctor said, "*Good*, Mistuh Dingle! I'll leave the form here so you can talk it over with your family, okay? We can come pick it up latuh."

Then, in a remarkable and rare display of compassion, she lowered her voice and said, "I know this is hard, Mistuh Dingle. It's a difficult decision." She turned from his bed and started walking around the curtain, past me, toward the door. Striding by, as if she just couldn't release herself from the last line of the pathetically predictable script, she called back, "Have a good day, Mistuh Dingle."

I wanted to leap out of the bed and tackle her. I wanted to grab her by the neck and strangle her. I wanted to say, "You fucking bitch. How dare you? How dare you wake this man up at five in the morning to give him news like that? Five hours before any visitors are even allowed on the floor to see him. And who do you think you're talking to anyway? That's Willie Dingle over there. Willie Dingle doesn't even know what a 'mass' is. He doesn't know 'extraordinary measures' or 'resuscitate,' and he sure as fuck doesn't know what 'incapacitated' means — even before you hypnotized him with the word. And worse than any of that, who do you think you are, telling him all that horrible gruesome shit *right here in the room where I have to listen to it too?!* You think I don't have problems of my own I have to worry about? You think I need to be here when Willie Dingle hears he hasn't got a prayer left in this world, and that no one's heard any of his prayers so far anyway?" I wanted to kill this doctor for her stupidity, for her insensitivity, and for her complicity in the conspiracy that had trapped me there. And I wanted to kill her for nothing more than being the messenger who had brought the bad news.

She smiled at me as she left the room and faded away down the hall. I watched her go and didn't say a word. I learned that I had been wrong about my neighbor Willie, and about what he could and couldn't understand. As the first rays of light squeezed through the break in the curtains, in the silence of the aftermath of the attack, I lay still in my bed and I listened to Willie Dingle cry.

The next day I moved myself into a private room. The cost was $150 a day above what my insurance would pay for. I never asked about Willie Dingle again, and I did my best to avoid even going back down to that end of the floor. Besides the arguable insanity of placing one patient preparing for a bone marrow transplant in a room with another patient suffering from all of the procedure's worst complications, I just couldn't bear to be around any more grief than my own life contained already.

There was also now a great urgency to the treatment schedule. The only hope for survival from that moment on was to get the leukemia into remission once more, to recover from that battle, and then to have a bone marrow transplant as quickly as possible. The leukemia once again proved to be highly susceptible to the chemotherapy and a second remission was soon achieved. But then one night, as I lay in the hospital counting the moments until I'd be well enough to move on to step two and wondering how long this new remission might hold, I got a fever. The fever rose that night to 106.5 degrees. The fever came on with the force of a storm brewing inside my body. A restlessness. An energy that was trapped, that was looking for a path to blow but that could only inhabit a tiny space and burn itself out. I would just have to wait. And wait I did.

For the next ninety days I had that fever. It would explode at two in the morning, then level off for several hours. Just before dawn, it would attack once more, only to drowse at mid-morning. That's when I would sleep, when the fever would let me. With a fever of such strength, but no clear diagnosis, the treatment is minimal. Tylenol is given every four hours. And when the hot winds blew, when it seemed that the apocalypse had arrived and was launching its mad fury from within my very own flesh, on went the cooling blanket.

A cooling blanket isn't really a blanket at all. It's a pad laid on the bed, underneath the sheet. The pad is hooked up, by thick rubber tubes, to a large machine on wheels, which, when turned on — besides causing a holy racket of whooshing, grinding, screaming sounds — sends jets of ice-cold water through the pad on the bed. This is done to try to lower the temperature of the patient, and it causes, much like the Shake and Bake I'd come to know so well, violent shivering spasms alternating with crippling heat and sweats.

For two months I lay on that cooling blanket. I was put through every test, every procedure that any specialist could have conceivably recommended: magnetic resonance imaging; radioactive white blood cell scans; liver needle biopsy. Some of these maneuvers were conducted using enormous, gleaming machinery. Just as often, they were performed in dank, grimy cells below ground level, with sunlight struggling to penetrate the filthy windows near the ceiling of the room. I saw the miracle of modern medicine revealed as what it truly is: an astonishing assortment of marvelous tools that serve only to practice a thorough process of elimination. With this lineup of equipment, doctors are able to look for clues in one area of the body and then continue to search in an achingly wide arc through the list of every possibility until they get a positive result. In the most arduous endurance test imaginable I was probed, punctured, and drained. Infused with gallium and barium. Twisted, spun, wrung out, and plopped back into bed. Every test was performed that was available, yet no diagnosis was found. As the doctors began to speak about sending surgeons to see me — surgeons who could offer me various types of exploratory surgery, as a salesman might offer samples from a briefcase — all I was told was that "fifty percent of the time, fevers of unknown origin are not diagnosed until autopsy."

In fact, this cold, detached casualness about my possible death had become the norm in the doctors' behavior toward me. While I had enjoyed a warm, if still somewhat formal, relationship with Dr. Melman, since my problems had become more serious I was detecting an undeniable change in her attitude. The amusement that she had at one time gotten from my breadth of knowledge about my illness, as well as her exasperated admiration of my logical arguments for altering some of the hospital's routines, had vanished. Her daily visits changed into brusque, rote reports that she would conclude with a shrug of her shoulders. Day after day she would stand at the foot of my bed and say, "I'm afraid we have nothing new to tell you, Evan."

I can't fault Jesselyn Melman for not having any more information for me. But each day would bring a parade of several different doctors and nurses. An intern would stop by, as would a resident. Every shift change brought a new nurse, and, in addition to whatever specialists might be monitoring my progress, once a day I saw Dr. Melman, my attending physician. Unvaryingly, the worse my condition became, the more curt and strained were their daily visits. It was as if these professionals, and whatever warmth they might have once shown me, began receding in direct proportion to how poorly I was faring.

Perhaps as a result of their frustration at having to stand by my bedside and continually confess their ignorance over the cause of my problems, another tactic became common. Some of the younger doctors took to bursting into my room with a bizarrely forced, cheerful demeanor, making pronouncements about what the next plan of attack was going to be. Apparently these people, lower in the hospital hierarchy than they wanted to be, needed to feel that they had some news item for me, because I counted six occasions, over a seven-day period, when I was told by a staff member that "they've decided on surgery for you."

I would explode when this happened, and the poor soul who had been presumptuous enough to utter the statement would gawk at me, puzzled by my anger. "What the fuck do you mean?" I'd snarl. "Who's decided on surgery for me, and since when does surgery get decided on *for* someone? Am I wrong, or don't I at least get a vote on the matter?"

"Oh, well, I don't . . . of course you do. I was just . . . it's just what I'd heard."

"Yes, well," I'd snap back. "Why don't you leave those discussions to me and my attending physician?"

"Of course. Of course."

But no matter how I complained, this happened day after day. I had agreed to have a surgeon examine me, and to listen to his recommendations. But why were these interns and residents and nurses parading into my room with news about what the hospital had "decided" to do to me? And what kind of staff did they have there, anyway? Who could possibly think along the lines of doctors deciding what would be done to a patient without that patient's prior knowledge or consent?

When I asked Dr. Melman what was going on, she seemed perplexed as to what I was so upset about. "Ignore them," I was told. But if a half-dozen hospital employees could, though mistaken, be certain that they knew what was in store for me, how could I rest assured that one of them wouldn't arrive before dawn, administer a sedative, and cart me away to the operating room? And if there was such efficient communication among the staff that everyone could share information, why was it impossible to replace the rumor with facts?

*   *   *

About the only pleasure I allowed myself during those two months was having my friend Daniel come and sing to me in the hospital. We had gotten to know each other about a year before, during my stay at Sundance Institute, and we had played around at writing a couple of songs together there. What that really means is that Daniel indulged me by letting me contribute a few lyrics to one of his beautiful creations.

Daniel is a born musician, from an intensely musical family, who writes songs of simple, elegant, inspirational beauty. Most are love songs, with a strong country/gospel feeling, and many invoke soaring images of faith and redemption. We had become fairly good friends since spending part of the previous summer together, and dinners with Dan and his girlfriend, Barbara, and Jackie had become a common occurrence. Daniel and I had begun planning a cross-country bicycle trip together, one that would take us from New York all the way back to Sundance, in Utah, for the next summer's session. I was taking particular pleasure from our girlfriends' vested interest in the trip. Apparently Dan's girlfriend had been getting annoyed with his stunningly self-effacing manner and wished that someone would instill a bit of assertiveness in her sweet-natured man. Jackie, on the other hand, had witnessed about all she could stand of my competitive, self-promotional personality, and it was clear that each of the females was openly coveting a little bit of the other woman's man, and hoping we'd come back from the journey ever so slightly altered by our exposure to each other. I suppose if we'd been thirty years or so older, some easygoing mate-swapping might have been the more sedentary solution. But being the healthy young bucks that Dan and I were, we all hoped our bicycling two thousand miles together might do the trick.

It was the casting of *Broadway Bound* that caused the cancellation of our trip. But we had stayed close and just a day or two after the new diagnosis, we all had dinner together. We met on the Upper West Side of Manhattan at a restaurant specializing in steak. I had decided to bulk up before I headed off down the road to Hell once more, and I remember gathering at the restaurant, showing them my Valium prescription, and working very hard to make heroic jokes about my plight. In the middle of a sentence I was speaking, Daniel reached over, and in an act of intimacy that embarrassed me to the core of my being, put his hand over mine on the tabletop.

"I'm gonna go through it with you this time, buddy," he said. "I'll be with you the whole way."

I nodded my head mutely and tried to blink back my tears. Daniel and Barbara had heard me, many times, disparage the friends who had "abandoned" me during the first episode of my illness. Friends who had faded away over the last two years, either immediately following the first diagnosis or somewhere else along the line. Friends who'd sent a card or bouquet but who'd never shown their faces or called on the phone. And I don't mean to suggest that I craved the presence of people I wasn't close to. I refused dozens of visits from distant relatives or friends of my parents who thought nothing of arriving at the hospital unannounced with the deluded notion that I would be happy to see them. An impromptu hospital visit to someone who is seriously ill is not, in my opinion, the way to demonstrate support for their family. I'm speaking of friends whom I saw or spoke to on a weekly, or even daily, basis, and whom I never heard from again.

Daniel cut right through my stoic posturing and spoke precisely what I'd longed to hear. That is something that takes an incredible amount of courage. The only thing that takes more is to live up to the promise. And live up to it he did. For hours at a time, Daniel would sit on the bright orange, plastic-covered, institutional furniture of my hospital room. I would lie in my bed, heavily sedated by pain medications, with several drugs and blood products at a time flowing into the catheter in my chest. After the recurrence of the illness, Dr. Melman, being diplomatically uncritical of Zweig's earlier decision, had agreed that it was time to implant a more permanent vein-access system. In an operating room procedure, while I was under general anesthetic, a small rubber tube was inserted into one of the major veins in my neck until its end rested inside a chamber of my heart. The other end was tunneled under my skin until it emerged a few inches to the right of my left nipple, where it branched off into two separate tubes, each capped with a rubber port for sticking needles into. This device, while gruesome to look at at first, emerging from my flesh like some two-headed parasite, would save me from having any more needles stuck into me. With scrupulous hygienic care this Broviac catheter could remain in place indefinitely. There was, though, a constant risk of a serious infection infiltrating the equipment, and, if that were to occur, I was told, the catheter would quickly have to be removed. I cared for mine as if it were a helpless creature, dependent on me for its life. Whenever nurses administered drugs to me through it, I would chastise them if they didn't clean the access ports adequately, and I would ask them to push their potions in slowly. This method of delivery resulted in almost instant effectiveness of the drugs, and, as was common, if the drugs were pushed in too fast, they would cause intense chemical tastes to flood my mouth and throat, as well as an overwhelming sense of nausea.

Half-conscious, deeply depressed, and severely ill, I was not a pretty sight or a pleasant host. Without the help of a major narcotic, Dilaudid, administered every four hours, I was in agony as the result of a severely swollen liver — the only diagnostic clue we ever got as to the cause of my fevers. Yet Daniel would quietly unpack his mandolin in the darkened room, sit himself down near the foot of the bed and begin to play. Oftentimes Jackie would climb onto the bed next to me, and in the only exertion of energy I might make for the entire week, I would softly sing along with my friend Daniel as he played. The mood in the room was hushed. Reverential. The degree of suffering being endured was granted an equal measure of respect. Panting in the bed, with Daniel singing to me and Jackie stroking my burning head, I had arrived at the place to which I had fought so hard to avoid falling: I was a patient. And there was nothing for me to do but live up to the label, to wait, and to accept whatever might come to pass. For the first time, with no strength left to struggle, I understood where the term had come from, and what it was supposed to mean.

At one of the bleakest points during the fever's sway, after all diagnostic attempts had proven futile by proving nothing at all, I was finally introduced to Dr. Gee. As in, "Gee, why didn't anyone think of this before?"

I'd heard about Dr. Gee since I had first arrived at that hospital. He was known as a "good guy." During each stay I made at Sloan-Kettering someone — another patient, a nurse — would ask me, "Do you know Dr. Gee?" When I'd answer no, they'd say "Oh, too bad. He's a really good guy." The only reason I hadn't sought him out as my own physician was that, at the time I was diagnosed, I'd been told he was too busy to take on any more cases. So when Dr. Melman started fortifying her daily bedside shrugs with a mumbled "Maybe I'll have Tim Gee stop by to see you," my ears perked up. Dr. Melman elaborated over the next few days, adding that Dr. Gee had greater knowledge of leukemia treatment and its complications than anyone else on the staff. If there was someone who might be able to figure out what was wrong with me, she said, it would be Timothy Gee.

I had become reluctant to have any new doctors examine me. Besides the fact that they each ordered a series of additional exhausting tests, the examinations themselves were hard to tolerate. In addition to having the undiagnosed fever, I was also in distress from various more easily identifiable difficulties. The most painful of these was a severe rectal infection which caused a burning ache to spread out from its fragile epicenter through every nerve in my body. I didn't want any more doctors to come see me because, quite simply, it hurt like hell to be touched.

Late one night, in the still hours after the rotting dinner remains had been cleared away, there was a soft knock on my door. I turned the volume down on the five-inch television set that was suspended on a retractable arm over my bed. If you've ever despaired over the lack of watchable television shows being broadcast, you can imagine how that despair deepens into despondency when left alone to pass another feverish night in a hospital room. Why cable TV stations like Home Box Office haven't worked out deals with hospitals is a puzzle to me. I can't imagine that customers of the medical centers wouldn't be willing to pay a few dollars more per day to have some additional options when it comes to whiling away long, and often frightening, hours, days, weeks. And if the cable companies had a drop more foresight, I think they'd find that a donation of their services to hospitals would lead to an increase in subscribers once the patients returned home.

Since the staff member who knocked on a door was an endangered species, and since visiting hours had long since passed, I couldn't imagine who might be waiting on the other side for my reply. When an extremely tall Asian man poked his head into the room and asked, "Mr. Handler, is it all right if I come in?" I recognized him from the outpatient clinic as Dr. Timothy Gee. Dr. Gee stood well over six feet tall, although his height was tempered somewhat by a marked stoop in his posture. With a friendly nod, Dr. Gee walked into the room and around my bed until his physical presence was as deeply committed to the space as was possible. He pulled up a chair, and he sat down to talk.

Dr. Gee first asked me to tell him what I had been watching on television. When he heard it was a ballgame, he wanted to know the teams and the score. Once he knew the score, he was curious as to whom I wanted to win. Dr. Gee chatted easily with me, in a soothing voice, before moving on to the medical matters at hand. Even after the transition to business had occurred, I found his demeanor to be exquisitely sensitive to the fact that he had come into the temporary home of another individual. Dr. Gee explained precisely what type of examination he *hoped* to perform, rather than planned to. He asked me how I felt about everything he proposed. Dr. Gee asked me to let him know if there were any areas that I was especially apprehensive about having examined, and he requested that I instruct him as to any ideas that I might have about what was going on inside my body. In essence, Timothy Gee invited me to participate with him in his investigation. Not merely to endure it. Not to make myself scarce while he had a go at my body. But rather, to allow him to try to help me by joining him in the attempt. This cultivated in me an eagerness to reciprocate the level of attention being given to me. Dr. Gee brought the simple principles of human interaction to his work. I don't know if his technique was calculated or intuitive, but he apparently understood that people are more willing to give of themselves to someone with whom they share a relationship, and that the quality of that relationship will determine the level of trust granted to the other.

Once the examination began, the obviousness of the differences between Timothy Gee's capabilities and the other doctors' expanded galactically. I was stunned by the disparity. When Dr. Gee touched me he was gentle. And yet, "gentle" is insufficient. Tender. That was it. Dr. Gee touched my body as he might handle something that was delicate and that was precious to him. There was reverence in his touch. And humility. Timothy Gee, from the moment he entered the room, made no assumptions of superiority and held no illusions that asserting it might simplify his assignment. Dr. Gee practiced medicine as if he were attempting to commune with divinity. He possessed the humbleness of one who wishes to be granted access to a realm in which there are infinite forces at work, most of them wielding powers much more marvelous than his own. Ultimately,

Dr. Gee had no more success in identifying the source of my fever than anyone else. But he succeeded in setting a standard that very few medical professionals I had met ever approached.

Even at the time I was aware of the idiocy in the fact that his behavior should be such a revelation, but the evidence was substantial. Such simple, sensible talent had been a colossal rarity during my stays at Sloan-Kettering. Not unheard of, but glaringly scarce. And I wondered why this was. Why for every Timothy Gee were there twelve Zweigs? How could thirty nurses whose most distinctive feature was their indifference share duties with the few who were truly dedicated? And what was it that set the devoted ones apart? Had the bad ones once been good, and, if so, what was it they had lost along the way? Inevitably, this imbalance results in the greatest battles being forced on those who wish to do the best work. Because each extra effort they make becomes an affront to the person who refuses to demand as much from him or herself. Thus, acceptance of mediocrity is quickly transformed into insistence upon it, and the message is clear for both the staff and patients: cooperate rather than excel. I have seen the same syndrome demonstrated in every arena I've encountered, from education to the entertainment industry. Even so, I was astonished to find that it was prominently practiced when the stakes were as high as life and death.

Karen, the nurse who had stopped by my bed to terrorize me on one of my first nights in the hospital a couple of years before, continued to visit regularly. I'd rail on to her about the way the doctors had distanced themselves as soon as they started to feel powerless to help me; or how it seemed like the hospital was designed for either quick recoveries or quick deaths, and that my lingering in limbo was more irritating to them than either one of those options would have been. I told Karen how I would listen to the doctors outside my room, as they laughed and agreed that since they couldn't find what was wrong with me, I must be pretending to be sick. I must want to stay in the hospital, because I was afraid to go home. When I would tell Karen that maybe I never should have checked into this hospital to begin with, she would say, with the same calm, disinterested tone that I'd come to expect from her, "Yes, well, maybe you shouldn't have."

I started dreaming, every night, about executing the entire staff of Sloan-Kettering with a machine gun, all lined up along First Avenue. I originally had that dream late one night, after, earlier in the day, looking up to find that the drug that had been running into my vein for the last twenty minutes was labeled with the name of another patient on the floor. A few nights later, I woke up in the middle of that same dream to see Karen, my Florence Nightingale from Hell, silhouetted by the light pouring in from the hallway behind her. When she saw that I was awake, Karen closed the door to the room and stood silently in the total darkness. I heard her walk toward me and sit down in the chair next to my bed.

"Do you think you're getting the right care here, Evan?" Karen asked. "Do you think you're going to get well in this hospital?"

I had never even thought to answer one of her questions before. But that night, I heard my voice before I knew that I had decided to speak. "No. No, I don't."

"Well," Karen said. "Then you won't."

I remembered her first words to me two years before: "Do you think you're going to die of leukemia, Evan?" And I realized what Karen had been trying to tell me all along. In fact, I was able to see that night that Karen, who initially seemed to be the most vicious of all the sadists in the pain palace, was the true lifesaver, the guardian angel, of that hospital. She wasn't interested in reassurance or inspiration. Karen's mission was to get the patient prepared to confront the realities of his or her predicament. She found the patients whom she thought could be saved, the ones who might look beyond one particular institution for their salvation. She hunted them down and provoked them. When they were ready to hear her message, she came to them, secretly, and told them, as she told me that night, "You're right, Evan. You're not going to get what you need here. Get out. Get out before it's too late."

When the doctors' faces started to look too much like hungry vultures to me, when they seemed a little too eager to get to that autopsy so they could find out what had been wrong with me all along, I checked myself out of the hospital to live or die on my own.

Well, not completely on my own. Jackie was there to take care of me. And when she had to leave the house, other friends would come over to baby-sit. For me. I was helpless and couldn't be left alone. But slowly, over the third month of its smoldering reign, with a halting regression, the fever began to fade. Now, my temperature wouldn't rise above 102 over the course of the day. That was like a vacation. I started to consider myself well, and I would load up on Tylenol and go out and try to participate in life. I could now be left alone at home, and I would relish my privacy, looking forward to Jackie's departure for an appointment or to see a movie with a friend. When the daily highs dropped below 101, I started taking my temperature every hour, trying to will the fever out of my system before the leukemia that was chasing me caught up and ended the race for good.

It was well acknowledged, by now, that while Jackie loved me dearly and wanted my recovery more than anything, my illness had become a severe burden to her. Her devotion had become tempered, and she had developed a hardness to my suffering, out of deference to her own, which she had never seemed to notice before. As I prowled around the house one afternoon, while Jackie was out, I poked into the room where she had been spending hours of each day banging on an old typewriter. There were stacks of pages piled on the desk, but I didn't need to pry very far to get the gist of what was being written.

On the top of the largest pile of papers was a typed monologue, to be spoken by a woman in her late twenties, who is the lead character in a play. The monologue was a beautifully written, heart-wrenching explanation by the woman of why she has decided to travel in the west after her boyfriend has died of cancer. The trip is one that they planned to take together, she relates to a man whom she meets on the trip, and after her boyfriend's death all the maps and camping equipment began to arrive in the mail. The woman in the play goes on to explain his illness, and how it affected their love for each other, with snippets of the life that Jackie and I had been living together for the past two and a half years.

I was discovering two things at once that afternoon. One was the devastating realization that Jackie had, for some time, been preparing for the possibility of my death. As I dug further into her fantasies, as represented by the play that she was writing, I could see how deeply she had been exploring her feelings of my loss already — while I had been fighting to remain alive in the next room. This felt more threatening to me than if I had discovered her having an affair with another man. That would have been something that I could have perceived as a temporary substitute for my presence. This felt to me like someone who had already replaced me. Someone who had come to terms with saying good-bye.

The other thing that was revealed was that Jackie had become one hell of a writer. Her writing was not only skillful and filled with emotion, but it gave the impression of coming from a writer who possessed a personal power, a strength of spirit, that I hadn't recog-nized in Jackie before. She had undergone a transformation of her own that I had been too preoccupied to notice until now, or that had been purposely hidden from me and revealed only in those pages. I got my first glimpse of it, in person, when I confronted her about the play.

I told Jackie that I completely understood her need to write it. I told her that it looked like it would turn out to be a great play. My only complaint was that I thought it inappropriate for her to be writing it in the home that we shared, where I was still struggling to survive the very illness that she had already sacrificed me to in her fiction. I explained my discomfort over hearing the typewriter in the next room, knowing that it was her imagined life without me that was being crafted and perfected.

Jackie didn't bat an eyelash. Her purpose had become as clear to her as mine had been for me over the last three months. "Then I'll have to move out," she said.

And then she went on, "That's what I'm doing now. That's what I do. I'm writing that play. If you want me here, then you'll have to live with it. If you can't stand it, then I'll have to leave."

And that's the way it was. I could only try to keep her play as far from becoming the truth as I possibly could.

Although I was skeptical, I continued to stalk the world of psychic healers in search of a miracle. I got another recommendation from my friend Didi, and she gave me the address of a man who lived just two blocks away from my apartment. My eardrum nearly popped when Didi squealed into the phone, "You're gonna love him, Buballa. He's *amazingly* psychic."

Jameson Coutourier told me to meet him in the back room of his crystal shop on East Fourth Street. The neighborhood, in the years that I'd lived there, had become a hub for purveyors of accessories for the enlightened. I imagined his store to be much like the others, with incense burning, and New Age music playing as an astrological lamp projected images of the constellations on the ceiling. After ducking through the hole in a chain-link fence, and then cutting across a playground carpeted with broken glass, I got to the storefront, which was painted with various mystical symbols and quotations, and I banged on the door. There was no answer. I banged, I pounded, I was about to give up when the door was pulled open by a huge man with an alarmingly red beard and an equally red face.

"C'mon in," he said. And he turned away from me and walked into the back room.

Following him, I walked down a narrow aisle that was formed by handmade bins constructed out of plywood that had been nailed together and painted white. The bins stood on the bare concrete floor, also painted white, on legs made out of two-by-fours, and they were all filled with stones, seemingly divided up by type and size. The pipes and electrical wiring above were exposed, looping and tangled with each other, and all, of course, painted over in plain white. The rough-hewn white boxes of rocks had prices scrawled with Magic Marker on the side of each compartment. It was the first no-frills, generic-brand crystal store I'd ever seen.

Jameson sat in a swiveling desk chair, and I sat on the edge of a very low massage table that was covered in ruby red vinyl. I wasn't sure what I had come to Jameson for, but Didi said that he gave incredible healing massages, so when he told me to take off my clothes and lie down, I wasn't completely nonplussed. As I lay on my back, stripped down to my underwear and staring up at the corroded tin ceiling, Jameson prowled the room and talked about war.

"I been shot. Been shot six times. But I can't be killed. Because I've got an Indian warrior that lives inside of me. That's what you need, an Indian warrior."

I started to think up believable excuses for why I might have to grab my clothes and go running half nude into the street. Jameson was between me and the door. I was waiting for him to cross the room and give me an opening.

"I lived in the jungle for eight years," he went on. "I been bitten by snakes fifty-seven times. Copperhead. Rattlesnake. Coral Snake. Moccasin."

I was looking around his room. There were pictures of snakes on the wall. Thin, torn, peeling pictures, taken right out of magazines and taped up by their corners. There was a wooden statue of an

Indian Chief, a quartz crystal hanging on a string around his neck. There was a very large hunting knife.

I was drawn back to Jameson's voice. What he said next soothed my anxiety and spoke directly to me. It seemed as if a message was being given to me from somewhere else, with Jameson as the conduit by which it was communicated. In the middle of his lunatic monologue, Jameson Coutourier spoke out loud a fighting technique that I had been living for years already. I couldn't have described it until I heard it. I wasn't even aware of it until he gave it form. But his advice, in his strange little rock shop on East Fourth Street, perfectly summed up what I'd been through for the past two years, and became my conscious battle plan for the months ahead.

"The trick is to let the venom in," Jameson said. He was standing still now. Not looking at me, but staring off, sadly, as if remembering the events that had taught him the lessons he was passing on. "Make it part of you. And when the bullets come, there ain't no way to dodge 'em. You gotta know that the bullets are gonna hit. You just let 'em pass on through. Then they can't hurt you. You gotta run and meet the bullets, then let the bullets pass on through."

This image was immediately branded into my psyche. I had fairly vast experience, by this point, in rummaging through people's muddled philosophies and picking out the nuggets that I felt might serve me. I was already applying the principle to my anticipation of what lay ahead for me as Jameson rummaged through a closet filled with junk. When he came back to tower over me, he was holding a four-foot-long sword, with a blade five inches wide.

Great, I thought. I can see the headlines now. "DISMEMBERED BODY FOUND IN EAST VILLAGE DUMPSTER." Then, a week later, the big revelation: "MURDERED MAN HAD JUST SURVIVED CANCER!"

Jameson laid the sword on top of my body. The handle rested on my forehead, and the tip of the blade dug deep into my groin. Jameson sat at the foot of the table, and he started massaging my left leg. He rubbed the same spot, the muscle of my calf, first with his thumbs, then his elbows, and then his heels. The pain became excruciating, but I put up with it, because Jameson said he had found "a blockage," and it was important to get the energy flowing again. I lay there, grinding my teeth, thinking, Hey, let him fix it. Maybe he found the blockage that caused the leukemia. Maybe Jameson Coutourier will turn out to be my cure. And, of course, there was still the sword. I didn't want to upset him.

Jameson prescribed a tea made from boiling herbs in water for several hours. The tea smelled like dead, rotting animals, and it tasted just a tiny bit worse. My apartment reeked of decaying flesh for days after each batch was cooked. But I continued to see Jameson and to drink the tea, because he continued to talk about venom and bullets and war. He told me stories about the Indian warrior that lived inside of him. A lot of what he said was pure madness. But buried within were small gems, flakes of ore with which I was confident I could build my own shield, my suit of armor. In the back room of that shop, where I never saw a customer in over two months, I was sorting, sifting through the worthless pebbles, mining for gold.

When I was at last well again, shortly before entering the hospital for my bone marrow transplant, I took a trip to California to see some old friends. There were large groups of people who, due to my preoccupations of the past few years, I hadn't been able to see very much of. In addition to them, there were a number of friends whom I'd been in touch with, but not since the recurrence of leukemia. I had been informed of their concern; I may have spoken to some of them on the phone; but mostly, I had effectively barred anyone from gaining access to me since falling ill once again. Besides the personal anguish over my prospects for recovery, I was deeply ashamed at my failure to accomplish the victory I had already claimed. Between my celebratory return to Sundance Institute, and the advertisement I had taken out announcing my arrival back on the Broadway stage, I had embraced my position as the unlikely survivor of the unsurvivable ordeal. In fact, at Sundance, as I took up jogging and logged in my two miles each day with the other fitness fanatics, I wore a T-shirt I'd had printed up before leaving New York. It was a bright blue, tight-fitting shirt, the better to show off my newly gym-crafted muscles. On the back, in large white letters, was the proclamation: "LIVING PROOF." My posing was intended more to help convince myself of my safety than anyone else, but seeing how much others were inspired by my victory was one of the major enduring inspirations for me. When all my claims were proven false, on top of my personal anguish and rage, I wore a blanket of humiliation. I felt that I had let everyone down by failing to achieve the miracle that had allowed so many to believe that miracles really do exist.

Although I had become pretty accustomed to the idea of the risks involved in the treatments I'd had and the ones I was facing, that doesn't mean they didn't scare the hell out of me. I was terrified. But it was much easier for me to broach conversations in which I would casually mention the 20 percent mortality rate of the transplant procedure than it was for my friends to hear about it. Especially friends in California who hadn't seen me in some time and whose only exposure to the whole mess had come from reports they'd gotten from other mutual friends. I called them all, one by one, and would meet them for dinner, or just to hang out for the day. I'd fill them in on the last three years of my life. Then I'd tell them how one out of every five people who check into the hospital for a bone marrow transplant never comes out. And I'd watch their faces change. And then I'd watch them realize that their faces were changing. And then I'd watch them try to change their faces back. But that only made them change once more, into something else entirely different in itself.

I actually had no idea what I was doing. I mean, I thought that I was just visiting with my friends. Just filling them in on what had been happening in my life. I had no notion of the burden that I was dropping on these people by encumbering them with such dire information in the midst of a jovial dinner. It was only much later that I began to realize how eager I was to share my load, how aggressively I was testing their reaction to my possible disappearance. Inevitably we parted all hugs and smiles, and I drove back to the place where I was staying, sobbing the whole drive home in the car by myself. Once I could see it clearly I began to refer back to that trip as my "farewell tour" of California. The most astonishing fact about it now is how well my friends all handled it at the time, one after another, right down the line.

Back in New York, on one of my last visits to the outpatient clinic of Sloan-Kettering, I was walking past the open door of the blood lab. I was thinking what a waste of humanity that hospital made me feel: sick people packed like rats, lined up to receive their painful procedures; all hoping that it might pay off someday, when they would run far away and try to forget it ever happened. I heard the bell ring and sped my steps to cram myself into the overstuffed elevator when, out of the corner of my eye, I saw a familiar face sitting in the chair of the blood lab twenty feet away.

Jesus, I thought. Jesus Christ, it's Willie. Willie Dingle. I couldn't believe that Willie Dingle had made it out of the hospital.

Just then Willie caught my eye, and he smiled. His eyes were clear and his teeth flashed a healthy bright white against his dark skin. He looked good. I forgot about the elevator and took a couple of steps closer, and we waved. I stood staring at him, just outside the door, in the hustle and the bustle of the crowd. I chuckled to myself at the memory of our cryptic, monosyllabic communications some months before. Every morning, the same lines. "Hey, Willie. How's it goin'?"

Willie's inevitable response had since become a favorite of my own. When friends or relatives would call on the phone to ask me how I was feeling, I'd get a private laugh out of adopting Willie's exhausted expression. "Ohhhhhh . . . you know."

I was nearly knocked over by a man on crutches who had bandages wrapped around his head. I caught my balance and saw Willie laughing at me as the blood lab technician jabbed a needle into the crook of his arm. "Hey," I said, grinning at him like a dope. "Hey, Willie. How's it goin'?"

Willie smiled a little wider. His expression was much more sly than I'd ever noticed before. He was wearing black, stone-washed, oversize jeans and a neon blue shirt and brand-new Air Jordan sneakers. I realized I'd never seen him wearing clothes before, nothing but a hospital gown. Willie sat looking up at me. He took a long deep breath, and he said, "Ohhhhhh . . . I'm pretty good, man. How 'bout yourself?"

ON BEYOND HYPE

While riding a train, I stepped out onto the platform to stretch my limbs at one of the station stops. Amid the swirl of passengers heading onto and off of the train, I glanced briefly in each direction, trying to form some impression of the land I was passing quickly over.

On one side of the tracks was an outdoor barbecue. A jumble of people in a dusty yard, milling about, or playing volleyball while beer sloshed up and over the brims of their plastic cups. A three-man band played twenty-year-old, second-rate rock songs as crusty-faced toddlers danced in drooping, muddy dungarees.

On the other side was an enormous field, broken only by the image of an old man and his dog. For every bit of random chaos that cluttered the scene across the way, here was only stillness and quiet. Suddenly, in one fleet whip, the old man flung out his arm, and out flew a red plastic disc. The disc floated on the air, spinning and sailing, never rising or falling in altitude. The disc traveled an impossible distance, really, as the man signaled and the dog took off in pursuit.

With wild abandon the dog ran. His paws pounded furiously on the grass and dirt. The man stood watching, himself as still as the rest of the field. With ears flopping and tongue wagging, the dog leapt and turned, snaring the disc in the grip of his sweaty teeth. The man watched, struck dumb by the sight, his useless body trying to comprehend how such a feat was possible. How anything could be so young, after he had grown so old.

I was on my way to Baltimore, to have a bone marrow transplant.

After a search that rivaled the International Olympic Committee's perpetual quest for the ideal locale, we'd set our sights on Baltimore, Maryland, and the Johns Hopkins Hospital bone marrow transplant program. Johns Hopkins was still having the greatest success that I was aware of with autologous bone marrow transplantation. And the statistics from their studies, while nothing to leap up and celebrate over, did offer enough hope to help me envision a better future — that is, any future. In addition, Baltimore was a city I knew and liked, and its proximity to home and friends made the move somewhat less daunting.

Jackie and I were traveling separately from my parents while they drove down with most of our luggage and their business supplies loaded up in their car. Once again my parents had halted their lives in order to help me rescue my own. Their efficiency in managing the swings between the tender calm of everyday existence and the frenzy of crisis had grown into that of a well-oiled, precision-tuned engine. As I had been forced to do over the past few years, with each new upheaval my parents would disassemble their lives to match the degree that mine had been shattered. Then, whenever time allowed, they would pick up the pieces and patch them back together, hoping that this time the glue would hold. Although I continued to carry a residual fury toward them, they only rarely complained, and almost never retaliated. Both they and Jackie had rented apartments in Baltimore, in order to be close to me as often as was possible. It was going to be a long stay, and my parents and Jackie were prepared to set up life in a new city.

A few years earlier, I toured in the play *Master Harold . . . and the Boys,* including a four-week run at the Morris Mechanic Theater in Baltimore. While there I stayed at the Belvedere Hotel. The Belvedere, at that time, was a grand old building, faded, but with an obvious glamour from days gone by. The hotel reminded me of an ancient, stooped old woman whose beauty is gone but can never be forgotten, due to her own remembrance of it and all that it once entitled her to. The Belvedere's lobby housed the Owl Bar, where one could still purchase a "yard" of beer, an old Baltimore tradition apparently, which is just what it says: draft beer served in a glass that's three feet tall. When the plans to go to Johns Hopkins Hospital for the transplant were finalized, both Jackie and my parents had, at my urging, rented rooms at the Belvedere. Since the manager of the hotel was friendly with friends of my family and aware of the reason for their stay, he moved them into spacious suites at no extra cost.

In spite of the fact that we were arriving in style, with fine accommodations and secure finances, we approached both Baltimore and the new hospital like a pack of skittish refugees who'd suffered for too long in too many different lands to ever let our guard down again. What we found there challenged our beliefs about the medical establishment, as well as our perceptions of ourselves as savvy, all-knowing New Yorkers.

The quickest way to compare the levels of compassion and humanitarianism of neighboring cultures, judging from what I experienced in New York and Baltimore, would be to visit their sperm-banking facilities. On a hunch, I had gotten myself tested before leaving New York and discovered, much to my amazement and that of several medical professionals, that I still had a viable sperm count. After four intense rounds of blistering chemotherapy, somehow my fertility capabilities were still kicking. Considering what they'd already been exposed to, this was like discovering that I'd originally possessed some remarkable strain of super sperm. Before checking into Johns Hopkins Hospital, I made an appointment at a Baltimore medical center and went to visit their andrology lab. This time, when I visited a woman in a window, I was given no small plastic container, I was given no thick manila folder, and no key. I was simply asked my name, very politely, and, after completing some paperwork, told to go into the room with the green light over the door. Once inside, I was to open the small wooden cabinet on the wall.

When I let myself in, I was amazed to find a spacious, comfortable room. The room was ever so slightly decorated, with a throw rug, and the main feature, one of those giant, padded reclining chairs. As soon as I opened the cabinet, I heard a bolt slide electronically into the door that I had entered through, and the green light over the door changed to red letters spelling the word "locked." In the small wooden cabinet on the wall was . . . What else? My little plastic container, with my name and patient ID number already printed on it. There was also a small, embossed plastic plaque that instructed me, when finished, to return the specimen jar to this cabinet, and then to leave through the other door, marked "exit." When I unlocked that door to leave, a flashing light would alert a technician on the other side of the wall to open the little wooden cabinet and retrieve the specimen. This done, the technician would replace the jar with a fresh one and change the light outside the room back to green, ready for the next occupant.

What a system! I thought. I was spared having to acknowledge to anyone face-to-face what was happening there in the room. The plastic container, the physical representation of the act, was touched by no one but me. It simply appeared and disappeared; there were no hand-offs. And the magazines! The magazines were in the room already, above the big recliner, arranged in a magazine rack suspended on the wall. Not arranged just any old way, either. These magazines had been arranged, on ascending shelves, in order of explicitness, with the milder ones in front. That way someone who wanted to look at, say, *Playboy,* but who would have been offended by something more graphic, didn't even have to glimpse the cover of the coarser material. How incredibly, how brilliantly considerate and civilized. The only way it could possibly have been more genteel would have been to serve tea.

The best part of the whole arrangement, though, was that when I left the room, when I left my deposit behind, I exited into an empty hallway that led right to the building's exit. There was not only nothing to be handed over and weighed, there was no one to face, period. There was privacy. After my odd, doctor-prescribed orgasm, I could leave with my thoughts and feelings intact, without having to cover them for any kind of social interaction. Thanks to their well-thought out plans, in Baltimore, once I came, I was free to go. Once I came, I was gone.

The storage fee in Baltimore was, and continues to be, a flat hundred dollars per year. In New York, the fees have risen to more than twelve hundred dollars a year. They started climbing after a lawsuit was brought against the lab a few years ago that was settled out of court with a large payment. A white couple had stored semen there and used it to get pregnant. Nine months later, the woman gave birth to a black child.

Returning to Johns Hopkins almost three years after Jackie and I had first visited and seen Dr. Rein Saral's "When all you have is a hammer, everything looks like a nail" credo, I began to see that every aspect of life there was infused with the same attitudes we had seen then. Even before our arrival, several weeks before my scheduled admission for the transplant, I received an information package in the mail. Included was a twenty-page document that outlined not only the treatment — how it would be conducted, and what to expect — but also gave advice about the lifestyle changes that would be necessitated by such a long hospitalization, and how best to cope with such things. The information included a telephone number for contacting the bone marrow transplant office and an invitation to call with any questions, large or small.

"They make it like going to summer camp," I told Jackie. I rifled through the materials they'd sent me, looking to find my equipment list, where I would be reminded to bring along insect repellent and a flashlight with extra batteries.

The treatment protocol at Johns Hopkins called first for a bone marrow harvest. To me, "bone marrow harvest" is one of the most precious terms any civilization has ever come up with. Referring to the marrow of one's bones as a crop to be harvested, the pungency of the agricultural overtones, evokes wonderfully homey values. The only thing missing was a wood-burning stove in each of the hospital rooms. In reality, what this meant was they were going to take me to an operating room, knock me out, screw needles into my hipbones, and suck out about a quart of bone marrow.

This was a procedure that I had already been through once before, at Sloan-Kettering. However, Johns Hopkins insists on using marrow that is harvested just a few days before transplantation. This, we were told, was for "administrative" reasons. Upon further inquiry we learned that by keeping stored marrow, the hospital was inviting the uncomfortable situation in which a desperate individual who'd stored marrow months or years before, but who was no longer a good candidate to survive a transplant, might plead for a course of treatment that now held little chance for success. By harvesting only those patients whom they intend to transplant immediately, they treat only those patients whom they truly believe will do well. In recounting to the Johns Hopkins doctors my harvest in New York, I described how the doctors there had removed marrow from the back of my hipbones; how they had then flipped me over and removed marrow from the iliac crest, the protruding bones that slope toward the pubic area; and they had then even taken marrow from the sternum, running down the middle of my chest. Using this last location, I had been told, carried with it the risk of puncturing a lung with the needle.

"The sternum?" said the doctor at Johns Hopkins. "The sternum? We haven't used the sternum since 1975."

So much for New York being on the cutting edge of medical advances.

After one day off to recover from the harvest, the drugs would be given. Four days of drugs would be taken in the form of pills, and then four days of drugs would be taken intravenously. These "superlethal" chemotherapy doses would effectively kill off all of my body's blood-making capabilities. Then, the marrow that had been removed from my body would be reinfused, just like a blood transfusion, to begin repopulating the bloodstream. This marrow would be first, with more metaphorical terminology, "purged," using chemotherapy agents directly on it to kill off any residual leukemia cells. If all went well, the "purged" cells would travel through the bloodstream back to their home deep inside the bones, where they would lodge and begin to reproduce. The reinfusion of marrow is referred to as the "rescue dose," which is appropriate, as without it one would quickly cease to exist.

An elaborate maze of euphemisms, to be sure. But they symbolize how at Johns Hopkins Hospital they are in the business, above all else, of trying to save lives. When I had glanced at my medical chart in New York — something that I felt afraid of doing openly, as if I were breaking some kind of law — I found within the two fourteen-inch stacks of rubber band–bound pages a completely different type of invented language. I read in my records that I had "refused" an unnecessary test, and I wondered why it couldn't just as accurately have stated that I had "declined" the procedure. I read that "the patient *denies* any unusual pain," and thought it sounded an awful lot like I was under suspicion of withholding information. When I read of doctors lamenting the way patients have developed "adversarial" stances toward them, I wonder if the origins of the adversarial aspect of the relationship can be traced to the language taught in medical schools. Language more compatible with interrogation than collaboration. And I doubt many of the textbooks have been written by patients.

When I showed up on the floor of the bone marrow transplant unit at Johns Hopkins Hospital, I found not a door with a number, but a door labeled with my name cut out of colorful construction paper. I was given a giant calendar for the month to hang on the wall, on which I was encouraged to record my daily blood counts and to cross off the days until I was well enough to go home — an active demonstration of the fact that the staff *expected* me to reach that milestone. I was visited — like a social visit — by most of the doctors on the unit, who would say things like, "I'm working on this service until the middle of next month. Hopefully you'll be out of here before me." When I would call for a nurse, the request that was relayed over the PA system wasn't "Jenny to 307," but "Jenny, Evan needs you." The treatment was still hell. There's nothing that anyone could do about that. But these people realized it was therefore a pretty good idea to do as much as possible about everything else.

From the moment that I checked into Johns Hopkins until the moment that I left; from the men and women who cleaned my room each day to the man who had helped to invent bone marrow transplantation, I got the impression that nothing was more important than my getting well. This was a teaching hospital itself, and it was a research institution — two factors commonly associated with the kind of gruff medical care that had offended me in New York. As such, the success of its studies determined its status, and so its financial future. But at Johns Hopkins, they seemed to have succeeded in understanding, and in communicating to the entire staff, that the way to get those good results was to treat each patient as an invaluable resource. That by helping each individual to *live* through the procedures, rather than put their lives on hold for the duration; and by encouraging and investing in each patient's recovery, they were enhancing their own results, and so their status in the medical community.

At Johns Hopkins all patients were encouraged — encouraged, cajoled, prodded, and pried out of bed — to walk twenty laps around the floor each day. One mile. I didn't succeed at it completely, but there weren't many days that I got away with staying in bed all day. It's not that it was so pleasant in the room, but going out in the hall required certain precautions and preparations. In my own room it was the visitors who had to gown up and wear surgical masks, but for me to leave, it was necessary to put on my own surgical mask and to thoroughly wash my hands upon returning. It sounds simple, but when connected to a rolling metal pole with thirty pounds of liquid and machinery, it gets tiring.

And, oh, at Johns Hopkins they had *great* IV poles! It was like they were ordered from a totally different section of the catalogue. These were sleek poles, with solid construction, that rolled and spun, and responded to commands like a fine automobile. At Sloan-Kettering it had been nearly impossible to find an IV pole with all its wheels working. These were the poles that patients were attached to for twenty-four hours a day, for four or more weeks at a time. And they didn't roll. So what they quickly became were shackles and leg irons. Any movement became an arduous task, and sitting still became far preferable to walking around. At Johns Hopkins, I decorated mine with ribbons and a six-inch Superman doll impaled on top. As I would spin around the circular track of the floor, my arm draped lovingly around my IV pole, Superman's cape would float behind us in the breeze. They rolled so well, those poles, that I wanted to organize IV races up and down the hallways.

And they had *computerized monitors*. For every fluid that I had running into me, I had a big, square computer box fastened to the pole that could be programmed to deliver the precise dosage, with an alarm that would ring if it stopped flowing. It may seem odd to get so excited about this, but all I had seen for dose regulation before were ineffective plastic clamps — chosen, I assume, for their inexpensiveness. They worked, clumsily, by simply squeezing the plastic tubing to slow down the flow of liquid. I had been treated at a world-leading, highly funded, and, I'd thought, glamorous institution. Yet here I was in Baltimore, Maryland, looking back on Memorial Sloan-Kettering Cancer Center and New York City as if they were underdeveloped third world bastions of neglect and deprivation. It was as if I had landed on another planet. It was, it still is, almost impossible to believe that two places so entirely opposite in tone and facilities could exist in the same universe, much less the same nation. And how had Sloan-Kettering done it, I wondered? How did they maintain such a renowned reputation, such a golden glow and imperious aura, when they seemed to relegate patient comfort and quality of life to such a low priority? I became burningly curious to find out how much each hospital spent per patient on things like IV poles, linens, exercise equipment; on anything that the patients come in contact with.

The differences didn't stop when it came to medical treatment, either. While I found the doctors at Johns Hopkins to be every bit as astute and just as relentless in their diagnostic zeal, they had one major advantage over the doctors that I had met elsewhere. They had no problem answering a question with the statement "To tell you the truth, I haven't got any idea about that. I'd have to check up on it." Sometimes they would even go so far as to say, "You seem to know more about it than me." And then they would sit back and start asking me questions, listening intently to try to learn what they didn't know.

I'm not trying to glorify ignorance. Not at all. But I had already learned to run away fast from anyone who claimed to know the most, or be the best, at anything. I had been told countless times by doctors in New York that seeking another opinion was pointless as, "we've got the best neurology department in the world here. If we don't know what's wrong with you, no one else will."

That's a load of shit, and in Baltimore I was able to see why. Down there they didn't try to convince me of anything, because they didn't have to. They had supreme confidence in themselves and were glad for me to check with anyone else, because they knew that I'd be back when I learned the truth. I'd come back knowing I was in the best hands, not because someone had screamed it at me, or threatened me with it, but because I had seen it for myself.

At first, all this love and kindness did was to scare the hell out of me. I said to Jackie over and over again, "These people had better cut it out. If everyone's gonna be so fucking nice and helpful all the time, I'm never gonna make it through." I'd only learned how to "fight" for my life, and I was afraid that if there was no enemy, then there could be no victory. I *endured* their affection at Johns Hopkins, while I waited for them to slip up and show their true colors.

It seemed that my neighbors in the next room had decided to solve this problem by fighting with each other. For two days, since my admission, we had been hearing the most awful yelling from the next room. A female voice, filled with such hostility that it was hard to believe she wanted any kind of recovery for whomever she was screaming at.

"Why don't you *eat it??!!* What are you, *stoopid?*"

All day long we'd hear this stuff.

"Enough already! You're making me *crazy!*"

A husband and wife, we decided. A special kind of affection.

On the day after my harvest, I stole my first look into that room next door. I was strolling the halls, passing time until Jackie and my sister, Lillian, showed up. The man was on the bed, flat on his back, with a tube down his throat, staring up at the ceiling with an incredulous and horrified look on his face. I couldn't believe that this was the man who was being screamed at so viciously every day. Later on, still craving my visitors, I saw a commotion from his doorway, and out came a stretcher with the man. His neck and head looked unrelated to the rest of his body, both in color and size. Still with the tube down his throat, he made a rough, gurgling sound. As he was pulled closer to me, his head looked like it had been inflated with a basketball pump. And his head was blue. Not a tinge of blue, but definitive and unequivocal. Deep and distinct. Desperately sucking on his rubber respirator tube, he seemed to be appalled that he was being forced to witness the beginning of his own demise.

A little later, Jackie and my sister showed up. I was never so happy and relieved as when Jackie would arrive when I was in the hospital and frightened. She had a quality of comfort that went beyond my powers of description, and an ability to inspire me on to deeper and deeper effort and desire. But no sooner had we arrived in my room, after my describing the morning's events, than the family next door must have gotten word of the blue man's death. The shrieks and screams of agony, disbelief, and loss — incomprehensibly irreversible loss — echoed through the halls. They epitomized all of my worst fears and fantasies, my most painful imaginings of control lost, and the grief of life and love left behind.

The next morning, after popping the combination of pills that would help to destroy my bone marrow, I was taken aback when one of the doctors said, "Why don't you go see the town today?"

I said, "What do you mean? See what town?"

"Go see this town," he said. "Nothing's going to happen here for you for the rest of the day. For these first few days we just ask that you come back here to sleep at night." And so, for the next four days, I had a vacation with Jackie and my parents in Baltimore. We saw the Inner Harbor area; we visited Baltimore's Little Italy; I'd go back to the Belvedere and take naps with Jackie. It was a great opportunity for us to experience some of the joy of life that we were working so hard to preserve. A great way for us to be able to experience each other as we loved each other before the coming days transformed us into ugly receptacles for suffering once again. Evenings though, became sad, as I would have to go back to the hospital and be left alone. Just as painful was leaving Jackie in a strange town to sleep in an impersonal hotel room by herself. I would watch her walk away down the hospital hallway, and I would feel her loneliness, and wonder why she would even consider coming back again the next morning.

*   *   *

Transplant day. With the toxic chemicals having poisoned the patient's marrow beyond any hope of survival, the time has come to begin the process of rebuilding and rebirth. A nurse is in my room. She is moving slowly, with a seriousness of expression and manner that renders the rest of us silent. The nurse is cradling a small bundle of white cloth in her hands, and she is handling the bundle oddly. Not in the shockingly casual way that blood and urine samples are tossed about, but with an equally troubling measure of exaggerated care. She steps cautiously toward the handsome young resident sitting at my bedside, raising and lowering each foot in what looks like a parody of someone carrying eggs over slippery terrain. Just before I make a crack about how she looks like John Cleese from the Ministry of Silly Walks on *Monty Python's Flying Circus* I realize what's happening. That is my bone marrow she holds in her hands.

Although it would still take several days for the marrow inside my bones to die off completely, the effective life span of the chemotherapy drugs is short. That is why the "rescue dose" of bone marrow, having now been "purged" of its transgressions, can be administered before the process of cellular genocide taking place inside the body is complete. Like an invading army, the cleansed marrow cells ride into a town that is still populated by natives, but natives who are doomed from their exposure to a weapon that has been sent ahead of the soldiers, that has sealed their fate and moved on. The occupying forces are free to enter and move about, to choose their new homes even as the former inhabitants are slowly dying off around them.

The preparations for the invasion to liberate the body are fairly extensive. Prior to the infusion of purged marrow, heavy doses of steroids are given. In the more standard version of bone marrow transplantation, an allogeneic transplant, a patient receives not his own purged marrow, but bone marrow from a donor. Even if this donor is a relative with identical genetic coding, there is still the likelihood of serious complications from graft versus host disease, or GVHD. This is a condition that is perfectly explained by its title. The "grafted" tissue, meaning the donated marrow, has no knowledge that it has been removed from one body and placed into another. To the perception of all the white blood cells that will ever issue forth from this new transplanted marrow, the body into which it has been deposited is actually a foreign force invading the body from which it was taken. To combat this falsely perceived invasion these cells will fight long and hard, attacking any and all tissues of the new "host" body, causing acute and chronic problems, which can range from painful and debilitating to supremely lethal. For some mysterious reason this syndrome is duplicated, in extremely mild fashion, in an autologous transplant, where the grafted marrow was removed from the very host it is placed back into. In this one respect, recipients of autologous transplants, such as I, face lower risks than those whose marrow comes from a donor. But since the risk is only reduced and not eliminated, the large dose of steroids is given on transplant day to try to control the reactions that are typical of GVHD.

In certain other respects, patients like me faced steeper odds than their allogeneic counterparts. First, there is a slightly higher risk of relapse posttransplant. The formula for how large a "cell kill" to go for when purging the marrow is both complex and imprecise. The presence of even one leukemia cell in the rescue dose can lead to a recurrence of leukemia down the line. Since there is no way to effectively examine bone marrow and be certain that no abnormal cells exist, the goal is to inflict as much damage on the rescue dose as possible without impairing its ability to regenerate. If the correct balance is struck, the leukemic cells, with a higher metabolic rate and weaker resistance, will absorb most of the poison and die off. Theoretically, the survivors of the purge will be the strongest of the normal cells, and, once transplanted, the descendants of these hearty cells will support the life of the host body for years to come.

Unless, of course, the marrow is so devastated that not enough cells survive to repopulate adequately. Nine days before, the morning after my harvest, a Dr. Barton had stood at the foot of my bed. He was a small man, with right angles everywhere about his person. He had a square head, with his hair cut into bangs that framed his face into a perfect box shape. His shoulders shot out from his neck at precisely ninety degrees, and his arms dropped off toward the ground to complete the staircase effect. He was a friendly enough guy, once you got to know him. But his manner was so crisp and staccato that it was just as fearsome as the information he imparted.

"Well, Mr. Handler, we got a reasonably good harvest from you and, I expect, an exceptionally good kill ratio. We hit your marrow hard. If it comes back at all, you should be just fine."

The assurance in his declaration helped me to feel very hopeful, and scared me out of my wits. I was terrified of becoming one of the people whose marrow never "came back," a dire situation that cannot be discovered until some weeks after the transplant occurs, when signs of regeneration are expected. I was afraid to ask, but I wanted to know if they had taken out enough for a backup dose — an adequate amount of marrow left untreated and held in reserve, in case the purged marrow fails to graft properly. This is obviously a measure of last resort, which offers little chance of long-term survival. The patient will have endured the risks and horrors of bone marrow transplantation only to wind up with the same marrow he started out with. But I was aware of one case in which a patient had to be given his emergency backup dose, only to recover and never fall ill again. The most likely explanation is that he was — of course, unknowingly — one of those few individuals who would have remained in a state of perpetual remission (another oxymoron) without any transplant at all. If you are getting the impression of a miraculous procedure defined by guesswork and imprecision, that was just the climate in the land of bone marrow transplantation in 1988.

Once I'd mustered the courage to pose the question, I was almost sorry I had. "Oh, we got a little left over," Dr. Barton announced. "Not very much though. We'll worry about that if we get there."

Sliced oranges had already been placed in dishes around the room. This was not to ward off or attract various godlike spirits, as it might have appeared to anyone stumbling upon the scene. The marrow infusion causes a ghastly sour garlic smell to emanate from the recipient for about a week after it's given. In the days before my transplant, we had walked the halls of the floor with perfect knowledge of whose had happened most recently and whose was some weeks behind. The smell billowed forth from the rooms like smoke pouring out of a burning building.

Jackie had already said good-bye and left my room. In anticipation of the horrible stench we'd sampled in the hallway, she'd given me one of our "noncontact" hugs, which were necessitated by my nonexistent immune system — both of us would spread our arms wide as if to embrace, leaving a space of two feet between us — and she'd fled the scene. Every now and then over the afternoon she would poke her head into the room, peeking at my parents and me, holding part of her shirt over her nose to filter the odor. She'd giggle self-consciously, wrinkling her nose up into an adorable attempt at a scowl and say, "I'm not coming near *you* for a few days!"

After I had been shot up with my GVHD-preventing cortisone, electrodes were run from various points on my body to a portable heart monitor. Since the infusion of marrow requires a large amount of viscous fluid to be pushed into the bloodstream, there is some concern about cardiac function. In other words, a heart attack is possible. If I was forewarned about the danger, I had no memory of it, so by the time the nurse arrived to actually begin administering the marrow I was in a state of high anxiety. The pomp and circumstance of what came next didn't alleviate it any.

As the nurse first unwrapped and then handed the doctor a large cylinder containing what looked like deep maroon sludge, I was somewhat baffled as to the solemnity being granted to the day's event. As I watched the doctor click the tubing through which the marrow would travel onto the first cylinder, I slowly began to understand the caution being exercised and the terminology I'd mocked thus far. The drugs had already been administered. Regardless of whether or not that marrow made it into my body, my blood cells were dying and there was no saving them now. As the nurse made her way down the hallway toward my room, as she held on to the cylinder until she was sure of the doctor's grip, she knew what she had possession of and the implications of what she was doing. I was in the same boat as the blood cells still alive in my body. I was a doomed man, and that was my rescue dose.

There were seven cylinders of marrow to be infused, and the contents of each one had to be pushed into my Broviac catheter slowly — over the course of twenty minutes apiece. It took me a bit longer to figure out the next part of the puzzle. Only after the first cylinder was empty of its contents did the doctor call the nurse back. And not until she took the empty cylinder from the room did she go to the refrigerator and remove the next one. If there were seven cylinders of marrow, I wondered, why had the nurse brought only one and gone away?

And then it dawned on me. If she took seven cylinders out of the refrigerator and tripped on her way down the hall, my life would be a gooey mess mixed with broken glass lying on the floor of the hospital. A maintenance worker in a green uniform would arrive with a broom and mop, and my life would be scraped up and cleaned off the floor, my only legacy a small island of linoleum left slightly brighter and shinier than the area surrounding it. Suddenly, the comical aspect of the event vanished and I was watching every movement the doctor and the nurse made. I studied her footsteps and projected her trajectory, ready to call out if there was anything blocking her path. I made sure the doctor squeezed every last droplet from the cylinders, refusing to relinquish my rights to as many cells as had been taken from me ten days before. For the rest of that afternoon this was the ballet that was danced on the third floor of a building in the town of Baltimore, Maryland. A woman wrapped my life in white swaddling cloths and, as if she were saving seven baby Moseses from the banks of the Nile, she delivered them to another man who gave my life back to me via a thin rubber tube. That's what is called a rescue dose. That is how a man is rescued, and that is how they rescued me.

On the fourteenth day after receiving my rescue dose of bone marrow, Dr. Andy Yeager waddled into my room. Dr. Yeager was a wonderfully odd little man. He was short, with a body like one of those Weeble toys that won't fall down. Dr. Yeager always dressed with a bow tie, and he seemed pretty thrilled with his work as well as his position in the general scheme of things. He spoke precisely, with great enthusiasm and warmth, but with the type of sincerity so rare that it provokes the slightest sense of suspicion — a bit like children's beloved Mr. Rogers on television. On this day Dr. Yeager seemed even more thrilled than usual.

"Hey, well, we're just, we're just tickled to death over your marrow, Mr. Handler. Looks good. Looks really, *really* good. Why, I might even go so far as to say, in an especially cavalier moment, that your marrow looks, well, positively excellent."

Andy Yeager had probably just added a good ten days to my ability to endure anything dangerous that might still come along.

Then he said, "Would you like to see it?"

"Wha . . . wha . . . what do you mean? Would I like to see what?"

"Your marrow! There's not a whole lot to see, we don't expect to see much on day fourteen. But I think I can show you — well, I'm quite sure that I can show you — some very beautiful red cell precursors; some very beautiful, very clear granulocytes in various stages of development; why, it's probably too much to hope for, but I could swear I even saw a megakaryocyte or two in there."

This had been my wish all along. To be included in all aspects of my medical care. To be included, so that, if I had to go through all this, it would at least be my journey and not just some ride that I was taken on, blindfolded, like a hostage. Now that the opportunity was being offered, I found myself paralyzed with fear. For the first time, I had an inkling of why so many people don't want the doctor to share too much with them. The reasoning goes like this: *As long as there is someone who knows more than I do, there is someone who must be more powerful than I am. If I give the doctor more power than I have, then the doctor will really have more power than I do. If I know everything that my doctor knows, and I don't know if I'll get well — then my doctor must not know either.*

I got up and followed Andy Yeager down the hall. I walked in a trance, like a medical student climbing the stage to claim his diploma, suddenly realizing that he is no more qualified today than he was the day before. Andy Yeager sat me down in a squeaky, wooden chair in a cramped, little room, and I peeked timidly into a microscope at the cells that had been taken from my body. He talked on and on about the slides he was showing me. At one point I glanced up and saw that his face was beaming with pride. When he caught my eye, though, his look hardened. He gave me a long, cold stare and, finally, gloomily, he said, "Well . . ."

Andy Yeager glared at me as if he was about to impart dreadful news. Just as my grin began to fade into a plea for mercy, his eyes brightened and a smile exploded across his face. "... what's your opinion? Doctor!"

I buried my face back in the microscope. I pretended to be riveted by what I was pretending to see, as I hid from him my tears. Tears of joy, cried over the doctor who let me be one of them.

The most brilliant illustration, though, of inspirational psychology at Johns Hopkins Hospital, in my opinion, was something called the "Evening of Elegance." I was told, upon my arrival, that each patient who makes it through to being discharged one or two months later, is entitled to an Evening of Elegance of his or her own design. This most often consisted of a waiter in tuxedo arriving at the hospital with a cart to serve a gourmet dinner of, say, filet mignon, fine wine, and something described as a "parfait sundae dessert."

It sounds nuts, but, oh, how that challenge takes hold. It's a fascinating psychological ploy. Maybe not for everyone, but it sure worked with me. I was not about to get cheated out of my free, hospital-supplied, gourmet dinner. For the next six weeks, through fevers and blisters, through emergency trips down to the monstrous machines in the bowels of the hospital, with mouth sores so severe that I couldn't swallow my own spit, I screamed in delirium at nurses and doctors, at my parents, at God and the devil himself: "FUCK you! I'm not going anywhere until I get my Evening of Elegance. I'm not going anywhere until I get my fucking filet mignon and my GODDAMNED PARFAIT SUNDAE!!!!"

When, at last, my Evening of Elegance arrived, Jackie and I were almost as eager for the dinner as for my release scheduled for the next day. The admission for the transplant had been relatively easy, lasting only six weeks — close to the minimum. Most of that time had been spent, to borrow an image used by airline pilots to describe their work, enduring periods of savage boredom, punctuated by moments of extreme terror. There had been a recurrence of the intense pain emanating from the area of my liver. Since this can be indicative of VOD, or, venal occlusive disease, a treacherous and often deadly transplant complication in which blood supply to this vital organ is cut off, the entire floor staff flew into action. With my father helping to push the gurney, I was again rushed down to the hell pits of the hospital to be scanned and, ultimately, reassured that I was not in the throes of my final campaign. There had been various fevers and painful infections and inflammations. But, until the night when I was scheduled to enjoy my catered party, none of the problems had proven to be as dangerous as we all knew they might have been. Most of my time was spent trying to amuse myself, sleeping for hours each day, and waiting for the weeks to pass. Then, as we watched for the arrival of our congratulatory feast, I started to feel a slight chill. As I wrapped myself in an extra blanket, the slight chill turned into a steady shiver. No longer harboring any doubt that I was heading down another dangerous road, I began to sweat, my teeth started to chatter like an industrial sewing machine, and my temperature shot up to 105 degrees. Clinging tenuously to the hope that I might still be able to have some sort of party that night and be released from the hospital the next day, I only realized after the dark red splotches began appearing all over my body and the doctors rushed into my room that after all the close calls and false alarms, I was in the midst of the real thing. This fire was worthy of five alarms, and I had finally stumbled upon one of the real killers I'd heard so much about.

One of the most common assassins of leukemia patients in the weeks following a bone marrow transplant is a fungal infection. The most common of these is Candida. A yeast. Jackie and I used to be endlessly amused that one of the most likely causes of my death would turn out to be the same organism that caused her vaginal infections. But, as all the lifelike color drained from my flesh, leaving only a gray pallor surrounding the now brown splotches; as the doctors pronounced my system to have "gone septic" with Candida krusei, there was nothing funny anymore about this tiny, deadly, fermenting agent that was running wild in my bloodstream. I was put back on the Shake and Bake I had become so familiar with, I curled into a fetal ball, and I didn't speak for the next three days.

Jackie described my reaction as if I had "retreated" into myself. As if every function that was not essential to the sustaining of life was shut down. She claims that I did, in fact, speak a few words to her over those next days but that mostly I lay very still, sleeping. Every now and then, she has told me, I would let out a sigh, or a slight, hushed whimper. Her parents came to Baltimore, and my girlfriend, my doctors, and two sets of parents held a vigil, waiting to see if the young man in the bed might pull through.

My only memory is of that first night — my Evening of Elegance — of turning my head on the pillow, too weak to even pick it up, and seeing Jackie. She was sitting at a portable dinner table, the kind with a hollow storage cabinet underneath, like those brought to a hotel room with a room service order. The hulking box was covered with a crisp white tablecloth, and there was a centerpiece of freshly cut flowers. I remember seeing her cutting her steak into pieces, and feeding those pieces into her mouth. She ate the meat and potatoes and dessert, chewing deliberately, squeezing the flavor out of each and every mouthful. When she had finished with her dinner, she reached across the table, and she started in on mine.

Two weeks later, after recovering from the Candida krusei assault, I was released from Johns Hopkins and taken back to the Belvedere Hotel. The treatment plan called for me to remain in Baltimore for a few more weeks, to be seen daily in the outpatient clinic, before being remanded back to a hospital closer to home.

The day of my discharge was a steaming hot, humid summer day. While I had taken a few strolls outdoors in the latter stage of the hospitalization, for the most part, I had experienced nothing but a filtered, air-conditioned atmosphere for two months. Since I was still considered to have serious immune system impairment, in spite of the heat, I left the building wearing a long-sleeved shirt, a jacket, a baseball hat, and a protective surgical mask. My fear over the contagious contamination of everything I might come in contact with had me wishing it was winter, so I could have added gloves and a scarf to the ensemble.

As we spun through the revolving door and into the lobby of the hotel we resembled an awfully strange entourage. My parents led the way, pushing the doors around, while I shuffled in my own compartment right behind them, afraid to even touch the glass. Behind me, bringing up the rear, was Jackie. She was making certain that the door didn't move too fast for me, that no one behind her sped it up to the point where I might trip and fall down. When my parents emerged they peeled off to opposite sides and flanked me for our trip to the elevators. Jackie burst ahead to hold a car, to make sure we had one to travel in by ourselves.

Walking gingerly into the lobby, wrapped like a mummy and skinny as a rail, with every surface covered so as to be nearly invisible to the human eye, I felt like Michael Jackson going into seclusion after plastic surgery. I wanted to get into the elevator and up to our room quickly, with as few people catching sight of me as possible. Barely out of the revolving door, though, I heard a stirring from my left and sped my steps only to see that the disturbance I had noticed was actually all activity coming to a halt. The desk clerks and bellhops, security guards and managers all stopped whatever they'd been doing and turned to face in my direction. I put my head down, humiliated, and wished that I could have disappeared. I couldn't believe that anyone, much less a hotel lobby filled with people, could be so insensitive as to stand perfectly still and stare at someone, especially if he looked like a freak. When I first realized they had begun applauding, I stopped walking mostly out of bewilderment.

Turning to face the room, an ornate and sprawling marble foyer, I saw the entire lobby staff, as well as many of the guests — some smiling and others crying — as they clapped their hands. The applause went on and on, while I simply stared back, baffled. I hadn't realized that so many people had been following my progress. I suddenly caught a glimpse of the lives my parents and Jackie must have led those eight weeks, surrounded by strangers, spilling their plight to anyone who'd lend a sympathetic ear. The anticipation of how much my journey back would mean to others, if I could make it there and stay, had long been one of the greatest inspirations I'd prodded myself on with. Seeing my fantasy so graphically displayed only increased my appetite. In the lobby of The Belvedere Hotel, I felt as if I had entered one of my fever-induced hallucinations while I received a long-awaited standing ovation.

DOWN TO ZERO

The completion of a bone marrow transplant doesn't equal immediate safety. The procedure is not a foolproof one. While surviving the dangers of the treatment itself is a large accomplishment, a full 50 percent of those survivors will again develop leukemia. The new wrinkle in this statistic, as opposed to the numbers associated with conventional chemotherapy, is that these recurrences happen rather quickly. Within twelve months, in most cases. While there are a few "stragglers," as I've heard them referred to, of those treated in the same way that I was, for the same disease, recurrences after twenty-four months are extremely rare. Those who make it back for their one-year, certainly their two-year, checkup in good health are considered to be "out of the woods," and in all probability cured of their leukemia forever.

When I first heard it, this struck me as remarkable news. With all previous forms of treatment, life had become a long, mysterious waiting game, with years and years of uncertainty ahead. The compression of the critical period was both a relief and a torment, as one might feel crossing the last hundred yards of a minefield. Safety can be seen. It can be imagined. At times it even feels as if it has arrived. Yet the chances for destruction remain just as present with each step.

Added to the heightened tension of the condensed time frame were the medical instructions upon leaving the hospital. My immune system would recover slowly, over the course of several years. For the first six months, I was strongly urged to practice extreme avoidance of all public places. No restaurants, no movies, no public transportation. I was told to avoid contact with children, with animals, with plants, and with soil. That I should share breathing space with no one who had recently been ill, or with anyone who had been around someone who was ill. In essence, I was told, for the next six months, "Don't go anywhere besides the hospital for your checkups, and unless you know exactly where they've been, don't invite anyone over to your house." The home stretch in the race to regain contact with the world required first that time stand still, while I lived in solitary confinement for six months, with no frame of reference for how long that was, or how quickly it might be passing.

Except for *Wheel of Fortune.* Two hundred and sixty episodes of *Wheel of Fortune,* to be exact. It came on twice a day five days a week. And it became my clock; it became my calendar. I've often thought, since then, of applying as a contestant, because I can honestly say that *Wheel of Fortune* helped cure me of leukemia. I've even suspected, at other times, that game shows themselves have curative powers. My association of game shows with illness goes back deep into my childhood, when the lineup of *The Price Is Right, Concentration,* and *Match Game Seventy-Something* would act as my nurse whenever I stayed home sick from school. The shows developed a comforting quality, as I knew when and where to tune in to find the same familiar faces that would help me to pass a lonely day.

But it was *Wheel of Fortune* that captured my heart. I suppose it was the lottery-like spinning of the wheel, which echoed the tentativeness of my own existence. Because even after the six months had passed, as I began to venture out — and as I tried so very hard to engage in life and to forget how dangerous the outside world had been for so long — I continued to watch *Wheel of Fortune*. I found, in fact, that I *could not stop* watching *Wheel of Fortune*. The treacherousness of that wheel — the cold, heartlessness of the black "bankrupt" mark on that wheel — now spoke to me in a language that I could understand far better than the one spoken by any of the people that I knew.

Due to the damage inflicted by the transplant, my bone marrow was unable to keep up with my body's need for blood cells. For the time being, until the marrow was sufficiently recovered, I would be dependent on periodic blood transfusions. But not just any transfusions. As a result of the frequency of other people's blood components being poured into my body, I had developed a resistance to most of them. As with constant exposure to a particular drug, the body's defenses learn to nullify the effects of any steady intruder. This was the same problem I had seen earlier in my old friend Willie Dingle. Whenever I was transfused with packages gleaming with blood cells that would once have bounced my blood counts off the charts, now there was hardly any rise at all. This multiplied the number of transfusions I would need dramatically — increasing the risk of transfusion-related infections — and so made it necessary to transfuse me with single-donor blood products whenever possible.

Generally, blood products, such as platelets, are composed of mixtures of cells from several individuals. Due to exposure to several different intruding organisms, this increases the possibility of rejection and of allergic-type reactions in the recipient. When a patient becomes resistant to transfusions, single-donor products are often tried. When resistance rises to the point where even single donors are problematic, sometimes the patient fares better with one or more particular donors. In my case, this turned out to be my mother and her sister, Bara.

Bara's platelets, especially, were like the Dom Perignon of blood products. Whereas a normal transfusion of mixed-donor platelets wouldn't even cause a blip in my blood counts, Bara's platelets shot the numbers straight up. This discovery relieved me tremendously, but, I'm afraid, caused Bara quite a bit of discomfort. Every third day or so, as often as she was allowed, Bara would troop into New York from her home in New Jersey to be drained. She showed up in my room afterward with her arms bandaged, sporting a fresh bruise from the latest needle. When the veins on the inside of her elbows eventually collapsed, Bara offered up her wrists. Although she never complained, I'm sure Bara had to be a little relieved when the doctors decided that, rather than risking my developing a resistance to her platelets as well, her blood ought to be reserved for any emergency circumstances that might arise.

All of these transfusions would be administered through my Broviac catheter, the small rubber tube that had been implanted in my chest several months before. As it had through the intense treatments leading up to and including the transplant, this tube offered direct access to my bloodstream without requiring a needle to be stuck through my flesh. The relief that this offered was enormous. During my sixty days at Johns Hopkins, the nurses had often been able to do their predawn bloodletting without even waking me up. They would let themselves into my room, leaving the door to the hallway open to provide themselves enough light, and then gently coax me onto my side so they could get at the little rubber nipples at the ends of the tubing. Like a sleepy heifer in the trusted hands of farmer Jones, I'd drowsily let myself be milked each morning. Milliliters; pints; gallons. They could have drained my body of fluids altogether without my ever becoming aware of it. The only thing that alerted me to the procedure was the chemical taste that would flood my mouth as the nurse injected an anticoagulant into the tube to complete her mission. This last step was necessary to avoid blood clotting in the tube and cutting off the easy access that was its very purpose.

As with many things in this world, however, such convenience carries its own risk. Easy access to the bloodstream for medical professionals means equal access for lethal bacteria. Many of the billions of organisms that exist on our flesh every moment of every day would be quite capable of carrying us off this mortal coil if they were able to gain direct entry to our tender inner parts. It's why you should wash your skin and dab it with disinfectant when you cut yourself. It's the reason why it's a good idea to spread some antibacterial ointment on an oozing scrape. The bacteria are always there, but we think about them only when we see the evidence of their opportunity. When we see what's supposed to stay inside coming out, we get the notion that something that's supposed to stay outside might get in.

Having a small rubber tube bursting through an opening in your flesh for months on end creates opportunities for even the most complacent of bacteria. The fact that the other end of the tube rests deep inside a vein at the entryway to the heart makes the pathway something more than merely direct. It makes it immediate. Add to the equation moderate to severe immunosuppression inside the compromised fortress, and then figure in the act of piercing the rubber ports at the end of the tubing several times a day — to pump fluid in or pull fluid out — and you have major infections waiting to happen. In fact, the patient who avoids getting an infection in his access line at one time or another is almost unheard of. That's why scrupulously adhering to safe hygiene practices becomes necessary. And after tenderly caring for my equipment for eight months without incident; after completing a bone marrow transplant, with the scent of freedom filling my imagination, I wasn't about to stop demanding ruthlessness.

Each day for the past eight months I had done as I had been instructed. After washing my hands thoroughly, I laid out a series of sterile packages. I carefully pulled off the bandage covering the site where the tiny tube poked out of my chest, and inspected it for any redness. If all was well, I opened the package containing the first of three Betadine swabs. These were very much like giant Q-Tips that had been saturated with Betadine, a powerful iodine disinfectant. The soft, wet head of the swab was then placed directly on the insertion site and, moving always outward from the center, wiped around and around on my skin in a circular pattern. The key was to never move the swab backward over where it had already passed. Any bacteria near the site would first be doused with Betadine and then moved away from the broken skin. After discarding the first swab, the procedure was repeated twice more. Once cleaned, the area was then coated with a small dab of antibacterial ointment and covered with a new bandage.

Besides the daily cleaning, each of the two ports that the tube split into had to be "flushed" every day with heparin, an anticoagulant. This is the same procedure that the nurses performed after every infusion or extraction, and it required its own special care. In probably the most crucial aspect of infection control, each time a needle is stuck into the soft rubber of one of the ports — an event that can happen dozens of times a day — the surface of the rubber has to be sterilized, lest any bacteria present be pushed right into the patient's heart and pumped throughout the body. Carelessness in this area can lead to an infection lodging inside the tubing inside the patient's body. Due to the extreme difficulty in clearing this type of infection, even with intravenous antibiotics, removal of the access system from the body altogether can be required. This not only increases the amount of pain and difficulty for both patient and practitioner thousandfold, but if the infection reaches a point where it can no longer be controlled, death can result. Mortality from an infected access line is not an uncommon occurrence.

In trying to minimize my risk of infection I had already traveled far and wide. Johns Hopkins insists that, as long as "adequate" care is available in a patient's home state, those patients seek their longer-term aftercare there. Limiting the patient load is one of the ways that the hospital is able to maintain the level of care that it manages to deliver. The first strategy was, immediately after completing the transplant, to move in with my mother and father. After our experiences in differentiating between the quality of treatment in New York City and just about anywhere else, we thought that the more rural approach of the Westchester County Medical Center in Valhalla might be a soothing alternative. The hospital in Valhalla had just opened a transplant unit, and I paid my first visit shortly after leaving Baltimore. Thinking that I had already seen most everything a major medical center had to offer, I was soon looking at Sloan Kettering from a new perspective.

In Valhalla, the doctors' offices were located in a different building from the blood lab. Since all cars had to be parked in the day lots, this meant that on the day of my very first visit, after having my blood drawn, I would have to walk a quarter of a mile, in the rain. When we arrived, wet, in the doctors' air-conditioned offices, we discovered that the hematologist I was to see, the man who was treating bone marrow transplant patients, shared his waiting room with a pediatric surgeon. After being told that spending too much time around a potted plant might be enough to kill me, I was sitting in a room filled with children and, at times, their pets. Across the aisle was the young brother of a patient. I heard his mother remark that he'd just gotten over the chicken pox. I nearly held my breath until we got back outside.

Since I would need a platelet transfusion, we then headed in the direction of yet another building, this one a slightly longer walk away. Something told me this transplant program had not been terribly well thought out. That was before I met Stu. Afterward, I decided that it had been brilliantly designed, if the intent was to end life as efficiently as possible.

Stu was the three-hundred-pound nurse who ran the outpatient transfusion facility. He was friendly, eager to please, and concerned about my comfort. And he was an absolute pig. Stu sweated more than any living creature I had ever seen, and he wiped the sweat off his brow with his right hand. His right hand, it appeared, also had a fingernail that was bothering him, because he immediately and repeatedly kept thrusting one of the fingers into his mouth, where he chewed and sucked on it. Stu put most everything else he touched into his mouth as well. The caps to the pens he wrote with; the pens themselves, which he gnawed like a giant starving squirrel; the wrappers to the tubing and needles, which he tore open with his teeth. When he uncapped the needles the same way, exhaling all over the one he was about to plunge into my Broviac catheter, I wanted to leap out of my reclining chair. The problem was, I was already medicated for the transfusion, with an antihistamine that acts as a sedative, and all I could do was close my eyes and pray that Stu was healthier than he looked. Once the transfusion was complete and I was back to myself, I stumbled out to my parents' car, drained and pale, where we drove away fast and never looked back. I went back to my apartment in New York City, and back to Sloan-Kettering, which suddenly didn't seem like such a bad idea. I should have known better.

"Are you trying to tell me how to do my job?"

"No," I said, lying. "I'm just trying to get you to clean the ports before you push the needle through. I don't want to get an infection in there."

"Listen, baby, I been doing this a long time. If you gonna get a infection in there, it won't be because of me." And the blood lab technician at Sloan-Kettering jabbed the needle through the rubber, after giving a cursory, glancing swipe with an alcohol pad.

At Johns Hopkins the blood lab technicians would scrub the ports of my catheter, first with alcohol, and then again with Betadine. The activity was done as if it were part of the serious task at hand, not an insignificant impediment to it.

"You better watch out, honey," I was told back in New York. "Some people don't like being pestered while they're working like that." The fact that her place of work happened to be on and inside my body seemed of no importance to her at all.

Within two weeks, I was in the hospital with a fever. The diagnosis: a gram-positive staph infection in one of the tubes of my Broviac catheter. This was the first infection I'd had in it since it was implanted nine months before. I was put on heavy intravenous antibiotics to see if the infection could be cleared.

As if this news wasn't dreary enough, I was told upon admission that there were no beds available on any "medical" floors, meaning floors where the staff is experienced in giving the type of care needed for nonsurgical patients. I would have to be sent, at least until a bed became available, to one of the "surgical" floors. In spite of all my experience up to this point, none of this struck me as anything to get too concerned about. I was well acquainted with inconvenience and figured that, by now, I could handle just about any situation thrown my way. I was assigned a room on the ninth floor, which specialized in neurological cases, and I headed up to do my time.

The seething madness swirling around inside Memorial Sloan-Kettering Cancer Center is invisible to most people passing on the street. The exterior of the building — the facade, if you will — gives no indication of extraordinary events within. Similarly, on a medical floor, while the suffering and deterioration of the patients is sometimes on display, their disease can frequently be concealed by the unblemished exterior of their bodies. Not so on a surgical floor. On a surgical floor, everyone's trouble has an image, and these images come in every shape. The shapes are formed not so much by what you see in front of you, but by what you know was once there and what is now gone.

The amputees. Human beings whose limbs have been expertly, scientifically, lopped off. They stagger through the halls, trying to teach their bodies to accept what their minds can barely grasp. Their losses are most obvious.

The add-ons. Their missing parts are signified by the devices that now adorn their existence. The urine receptacle; the colostomy bag. The hand-held electronic tool through which someone will learn to speak. Each piece of masterfully designed hardware acts as a confession. The indisputable evidence that at least a pound of flesh, once hidden deep inside, has been taken away.

And then there are the neurologics. The reconstructed contours of their misshapen heads are often the most graphic portraits of the human ability to wound in the pursuit of making well. Nowhere else on the body, even with the missing limb, is alteration from the expected form more startling. The graceful curve of a skull that now drops off like a cliff, as if some giant creature had taken a hefty bite. The luminous symmetry of forehead, one side of which has become sunken, like an apple left too long on the ground beneath the tree. These people, even if their brain functions remain intact, are branded with a physical imbalance. The precision of our bodies, which we depend on to reassure us that all is well planned and taken care of, has been removed, and what is left is something lopsided. An unwelcome reminder of the randomness that threatens us all.

On the ninth floor of Sloan-Kettering I was informed that there was a problem with the plumbing. There was no hot water available, and the cold water came out of the tap nearly black. Since extra-vigilant hygiene practices were of utmost importance in my precarious condition, this made for an inauspicious beginning. Brushing my teeth and bathing several times a day was looking like an over-whelming proposition.

Since the nurses were unfamiliar with most of the drugs I was prescribed, I had to maintain an extra level of watchfulness over their administration. Some of the antibiotics, when combined with other drugs, would coagulate in the clear plastic tubing that led toward my veins. The two colorless liquids would, if brought into contact with each other, form a curdled, cottage cheese–like substance that was rendered useless, not to mention disgusting, by the transformation. Each time nurses came to hang one of these medications on my IV pole, I had to remind them to change the tubing if the other fluid had been run through it previously. Many of the staff were unappreciative of my "interference," but if I kept quiet, or if I was asleep, often times a mistake was made, which set back everyone's already overcrowded schedule. As was the case with anyone in the hospital who upset the routine by making unusual demands on an overburdened staff, I was not the ninth floor's most popular patient.

My first night there, I woke up suddenly to the sound of liquid being suctioned through a vacuum hose. Like the sound of the plastic straw a dentist hooks over your teeth and under your tongue to suck up your spittle while he drills away. There was the muffled gurgling of a human voice, like an animal being strangled. I heard other voices, clear of congestion, hushed but intense, and there was a light on in the other half of the room. Not knowing how to escape or where I might hide, next I heard the sound of my mother cutting up a whole chicken into pieces for frying. The decisive grinding crunch of metal on bone, then the more extended tearing, snapping sound, as the leg is separated from the thigh, the wing wrenched away from the breast. I saw the larger-than-life-size shadows of two gowned figures, instruments in hand, hunched over a bed frame, displayed on the pale blue curtain that hung between them and me. I hid under the covers, afraid that this was a standard ninth-floor strategy. Afraid my turn might be next.

I had seen enough, I decided. My eyes could tolerate no more visions of horror, and my ears could accept no more sounds of suffering. I wasn't ready to die. I had no intention of giving up my life. Yet I felt I could not endure another moment of that existence, and so I concluded the time had come for me to lose my mind. If I could just get my brain to let go, I thought, then I could let all the agony around me fade away by loosening whatever screws bolted my awareness to the reality of my circumstances. I lay quietly in that bed, with my eyes closed, and — as the giant shadows chopped up the body on the other side of the curtain — I tried with all my might to go mad.

What I learned that night was that there were limits to my ability to manipulate my mental state. Although I tried, I prayed, I begged, and I cried, my mind simply would not let go. It was as if my connection to rational thought was an unbreakable bond. It was as if there was no bond at all, but that my mind and pragmatic thinking were of the same substance. I exhausted myself first with the effort, and then with my disappointment over my inability to sever my connection to the state of consciousness. In the morning, the head that lay attached to the body in the other bed was mummified in bright white bandages. It was two days more before I was transferred to another floor. I never saw it move, and I never heard it speak again.

*　　*　　*

In his classic novel Joseph Heller writes, "There was just one catch . . . and that was Catch-22." The predicament I found myself in next would have to be classified as a Catch-33, maybe Catch-44. Many of the drugs used to combat infections, whether bacterial, fungal, or viral, are also toxic to the bone marrow. Since the reason I had an infection was that my bone marrow was not producing enough effective infection-fighting cells, the necessity of taking those drugs only increased the asperity of my problems. As I was put first on intravenous antibiotics for the staph infection, then on intravenous acyclovir, an antiviral drug for the herpes zoster (shingles) infection that cropped up, my blood counts plummeted to nearly nothing at all, leaving me, once again, neutrapoenic, and utterly defenseless. But, thinking I had checked myself into the hospital for just that reason, to be protected against that which I was threatened by, I expected to hear the gears click in and see the life-saving machinery go to work. Not exactly.

Day after day the Broviac catheter continued to culture positive for gram-positive staph. It was quickly determined that the infection was not being cleared by the antibiotics and that the device should be removed from my body as soon as possible. Otherwise, the infection was likely to spread, leading to a systemic sepsis that very often results in death. The only difficulty here was that "as soon as possible" was taking an awfully long time to come around.

Twenty-four hours passed after the decision to pull the catheter was made. No surgeon appeared in my room. Forty-eight hours passed. No surgeon. Seventy-two hours passed, and I lay in bed, sick with fever, with infected rubber tubing resting in one of the chambers of my heart, and still no sign of a surgeon to pull the poisonous serpent out of my body. I was ready to explode.

Each day Dr. Melman made a visit to my bedside. She assured me that the surgeons were aware of the situation, and that, eventually, one of them would come up to the room and remove the infected catheter. She stated that I was in no danger from waiting "a couple of days," and she told me that the surgeons were very busy people who performed this procedure only when they found the free time after or between their operating room activities. Whenever Jesselyn Melman left my room, she was immediately replaced, like air rushing back into a just-opened canister of tennis balls, by several nurses who were checking to make sure that the tubing had finally been removed. When these nurses saw the two reptilian rubber heads still poking through my flesh, their faces tautened like actors pretending to be generals convening in a war room. They looked at me, and then each other, with expressions that I had seen before only in movies, as the portly gentlemen waited tensely to see if the errant missiles heading toward enemy territory could be called back. Olivia was often there. Gisella, too. And, of course, there was Karen. These were nurses who came to check on my condition even though I was no longer their patient. They stopped in from other floors on their way home or before beginning their shift in the outpatient clinic. The three or four nurses who, over the years, had proven to be unafraid of criticizing, or even crossing, the hospital when it was failing to provide the necessary assistance to their cavalric crusade.

Late on the second day of no surgeon I was in my room, surrounded by my coterie of professional advisers. By this time I had come to trust Karen to a degree beyond any of the other nurses. While some of them had aided and abetted my schemes to bypass the crowds in the outpatient clinic, and several of them had listened sympathetically to my complaints about some of the more egregious offenses committed during my internments, Karen had remained the only nurse whose honesty outstripped even her compassion. I knew that Karen would sooner scare me to death than let a lack of information kill me. When she spoke, it wasn't that she delivered any different facts from the others, but, rather, she sent a message along with her data.

"Evan," Karen said firmly. She held my eyes with hers. "That thing should come out. Now."

I didn't need to be told any more. With Karen's tone of voice illuminating her choice of words, I knew that I was being told that whatever I wanted from this world, it was up to me to make it happen. I waited for Jesselyn Melman to show her face again, and, although convinced I was in it already myself, I prepared to raise a little bit of Hell.

"Evan," Dr. Melman said to me, exasperated. "There is nothing more I can do." Our interactions with each other had deteriorated drastically as of my return from Baltimore. I hid from her none of my disdain for the lackadaisical practices of the New York hospital, and my attempts to disguise my abhorrence of her unwillingness to assist me in circumventing them were unsuccessful. I complained bitterly to Dr. Melman about the fact that it had been three full days since a decision was made that it was medically necessary to remove an infected catheter from my chest, and yet the catheter still remained. I wasn't dangerously ill at this point, but there was an active infection in the tubing, which was not being eradicated by antibiotics. The risk of the infection spreading and raging out of control was constant. Why was it still in my body? I demanded to know. And how long would I have to wait, how sick would I have to get, before it came out?

"The surgeons will come when they can," was all that I was told.

"Well, what if my infection gets worse and I die before they find the time?" I asked.

"It is my opinion," Dr. Melman said, "that you are in no immediate danger. Your condition is stable, and I see no reason to expect it to deteriorate."

"But certainly," I countered, "you have seen patients die from infected catheters."

"Yes. Yes, I certainly have."

"And you wouldn't argue that, in terms of risk reduction, the sooner the catheter is removed, the less chance of deterioration there would be?"

"Yes, I would agree with that."

"Then how can I accept just sitting here, waiting, while the odds of my situation are slipping steadily out of my favor?"

Dr. Melman became angry. I had seen her annoyed before. I had seen her lose her patience. But this was the closest I ever saw her come to losing her temper. She snapped at me.

"Evan, the surgeons are on their feet twelve hours a day in the operating room. I have told them to come when they can, and when they can, they will. I know you don't think the care you're getting is very good, but I believe that you are getting adequate care, and I can't very well drag a six-foot three-inch surgeon up here against his will."

I felt like the prosecuting attorney who has his witness on the run. I didn't think that Jesselyn Melman considered me to be in danger. If I was, then she might have dragged the surgeon up herself. But I also didn't want to have to reach a level of danger before anyone took appropriate action, and I told her so. I might be getting "adequate" care, as she said, but just barely, and certainly nothing more. And I thought that, on the other side of the company line she was toeing, Jesselyn Melman agreed with that and was angry at me for pointing out her hypocrisy.

"Dr. Melman," I asked. "What is the recommended action for an infected catheter?"

"If the infection can't be cleared, Evan, then the catheter should be removed."

"And if the infection is not cleared and the catheter is not removed, that could be a dangerous situation. Am I right?"

"Theoretically, yes. Of course."

"So, if I have an infected catheter, and it's been three days, and it hasn't been removed, and you can't give me a date and a time when it will be, how is it that I'm receiving adequate care?"

"You are receiving adequate care, Evan," I was told. "Because this is the best care that the hospital can give you."

It was the purest doublespeak I had ever encountered outside the pages of George Orwell's book. I think it would have mesmerized the inventor of the term himself. I felt I had been quoted a credo that granted anyone who really believed it a wide license to kill. But I never thought Dr. Melman really ascribed to it herself. I can only guess, but I choose to believe that Jesselyn Melman was embarrassed by the statement, and that's why, the next day, only four days too late, a surgeon arrived in my room. With a hard yank he pulled the dripping tube from my chest, and I tried once again to rest easy, trusting that I had surmounted the last obstacle on the road to my recovery.

The staph infection required that I remain hospitalized for at least two weeks while antibiotics were dripped into my arm. I would stand at the window, my forehead leaving greasy circles on the glass, and stare out over the East River. At night, lights would sparkle below, from the highway, the buildings, and the boroughs beyond. I would watch the cars pulsing like corpuscles through a vein as they crossed over the Fifty-ninth Street Bridge. I wondered who the people were, traveling away from this place where I was trapped, and if they had any idea how lucky they were. I wished that I could locate one single memory of what it felt like to be free, riding in a car, driving over a bridge, leaving something, anything, behind.

My blood counts, already at dangerously low levels, continued to drop. Neither of the bone marrow toxic drugs I was on could be discontinued — or "d.c.'d," in hospital parlance — until there was complete certainty that both of the active infections had been eradicated. The three brightly colored paper warning signs were once again posted on the door to my room, warning all visitors and staff members that the patient within was under "protective isolation" and that neutrapoenic precautions had to be taken upon entering. All who entered the room were now required to don a yellow paper gown and a surgical mask and to thoroughly wash their hands before coming near me. No physical contact was permitted, unless it was to administer medical care, and even then the provider had to be wearing rubber gloves. I had been in this place many times before but I had not expected to visit it again.

Next to my room was another private room with a similar set of instructions. Inside that room was a patient with pneumonia, probably the most fearsome and lethal of the possible complications. Every time I coughed or complained of anything resembling a shortness of breath my chest was X-rayed, to make sure that no bacteria were colonizing in my lungs. When a patient did get pneumonia, he or she was immediately placed in a private room, in isolation, but this time designed to keep them from infecting the other patients throughout the building. A hospital is the easiest place in the world to cultivate an epidemic.

It didn't take me long to realize that some of the nurse's aides who came directly from this room next door — to take my temperature every four hours, to record my pulse and blood pressure, to fill my water pitcher — were not gowning up upon entering. I saw them come out of the room with pneumonia, peel off the protective garb they wore in there, breeze into my room, and shove a thermometer into my mouth. They would clutch my wrist as they counted my heartbeats, wrap the cuff around my arm to record my blood pressure, make their notes on my chart, and float back out the door. I made sure to ask a few of the doctors just what precautions should be taken before entering my room and, upon hearing what I already knew, I started to complain to the workers who wouldn't comply.

"Oh, no," I was told. "You've got it wrong, honey. I only have to do that stuff if I'm touching you."

If I pressed the point, or indicated that they were, indeed, touching me when they entered, I got stiffer resistance.

"Listen, I just got undressed from in there. I can't be putting those things on and off all day," was a typical response. I began wondering if some of these nurse's aides had been trained by Stu, my three-hundred-pound friend from Westchester County.

Meanwhile, Jackie had been taking more and more time off to be on her own. The degree to which she had previously been sacrificing her own life was staggering, and, with my encouragement, she now came later in the day to the hospital, and stayed much shorter hours. It was no longer unusual for her to skip some days altogether. Her independence was something we both agreed could only be for the good, but it did leave me much more lonely, and it meant I would have to become better at fending for myself. In becoming my own guardian, I demanded the same conscientiousness I was insisting on from those around me.

228

I started to check the information being recorded in my chart. By this time, I could usually give a remarkably accurate estimation of my own body temperature, without the help of any devices. I knew when my temperature was normal, I could feel a fever beginning to brew, and once it clicked in I could count off the numbers as I started to cook. The information in the chart was not matching what I knew to be true.

Ordinarily, this wasn't a problem. Under normal circumstances, electronic fever thermometers are used. One instrument is used by patient after patient, with only a plastic sleeve being discarded and replaced between each use. The machine gives a short beep after about thirty seconds, and a bright digital readout of an accurate temperature, down to a tenth of a degree. But, under neutrapoenic precautions, the patient is issued his own glass thermometer, which is kept at the bedside in a glass of alcohol. As the nurse's aides came in and out of my room, blithely recording temperatures well below normal while I sweated through my bedclothes, the reason for the discrepancies I was experiencing became clear. The glass thermometer was being left in my mouth for the same thirty seconds as was required by the electronic one.

The nurse's aides' lackadaisical performance may seem trivial, but in postchemotherapy care, with an immunosuppressed patient, the fever chart is the map that holds all the clues. It is the first document that each and every doctor consults, and all decisions spring forth from the information recorded there. If a fever is present, then blood cultures must be drawn to find its cause. Once the cause is known, an informed choice can be made on how to treat it. If the information shows that no fever is present, then the patient is considered to be stable, and no treatment is prescribed. With a neutrapoenic patient, this disparity between information recorded and reality can rapidly become disastrous. If an infection, even a seemingly mild one, gets a head start on the medications, it can easily rage out of control. These dangers are exacerbated by the fact that, as I was to discover, the numbers in the chart are often given much more credibility than anything the patient might have to say. Doctors are seemingly trained to give all their confidence to the floor staff and their instruments, while maintaining a hefty skepticism toward their customers.

"Well, Mr. Handler. Everything looks great. We should be able to let you go home soon."

"Really? That's funny, I don't really feel very well. I think I've got a fever."

"Nope. No fever here, take a look for yourself."

"Yeah, but I *feel* like I've got a fever. I mean, I *must* have a fever."

"You're probably just anxious about leaving the hospital after a long stay. We'll keep an eye on you for another day or so, and you should be just fine."

It would have helped if the eye being used was kept open. I took to taking my own temperature immediately after the "official" one was recorded, and, sure enough, where I saw written 97.9, I registered 99.5. When theirs reached 99.4, I was really up to 101. Again, I asked the doctors to clarify the official policy for me. How long, I asked, should a glass thermometer be left under a patient's tongue to gather a precise reading of body temperature? Although it required some discussion amongst themselves, they ultimately agreed on a figure of at least four minutes. Judging from the response of the nurse's aide I told this to, I might as well have told her that she would have to strip naked and dance for me each time she took my temperature.

"Four minutes?" she cried. "Four minutes? I'm not staying in here for four minutes!"

I kept my own fever chart. It wasn't until I insisted that they take blood cultures that another infection was diagnosed, and it wasn't until the diagnosis that my statistics were believed. Once the truth of the situation became clear, however, the solution was just as insane as the problem. Rather than instructing the staff on how to properly perform their tasks and insisting that they comply, they asked me to continue to monitor myself. When I recorded a fever,

I was assured, a doctor would be called, and blood cultures would be drawn. Just as well, I supposed. I wasn't about to trust anyone else at that point anyway.

*   *   *

Dr. Sheldon Bimberg bounded into the room. Dr. Bimberg was a giant man, tall and broad, who gave the impression that his borders were intent on a continued expansion. Long before a movie was made of *The Flintstones,* in my casting portfolio, Sheldon Bimberg had been slated to play Fred.

I had never chosen Sheldon Bimberg as my physician. Just as, when buying a car, one cannot get the air-conditioning without purchasing the floor mats, he came as part of the dealer package. After establishing my early relationship with Dr. Melman, after initially becoming comfortable with her, and she with me, I was informed that they had gone into business together. They would share patients, I was told, and they would alternate, month by month, between the inpatient and outpatient duties. It was the last week of the month when this plan was revealed to me, and I was already scheduled for a stay in the hospital. The next week I would have a new doctor, and from that point on, the doctor I saw — either the one I'd chosen, or the one I'd had thrust upon me — would be decided on by the calendar, and nothing more. Someone should have handed me another informed consent form to read, this time outlining the risks and possible side effects of dealing with Sheldon Bimberg.

Since there was serious concern over the precipitous drop in my blood counts, a bone marrow aspirate had been taken earlier in the day to investigate the cause. Given the fact that I had just received a bone marrow transplant a few months before, recurrent leukemia, while utterly catastrophic, would not have been a statistically surprising development.

We had been through this countless times before. Jackie and I, my family and friends. A doctor would come early in the day, suck some bone marrow out of my body, and disappear with the slides.

231

As had happened on that day long ago with Dr. Nixon, we would then have to wait. We had waited outside Dr. Nixon's office, on that day that was remembered more like a legendary story I'd been told rather than as an actual event from my own existence, for more than three hours. Back then, we'd had no notion of what we were waiting for. Our faces had twisted into grotesque attempts at smiles as we'd joked and teased each other, our own creeping terror the only clue to what level of solemnity might be called for.

Since then, waiting for the results of a bone marrow aspirate had become an occasional, but somewhat routine, trial. We would try to amuse and distract each other as hour after hour passed. No matter how strained our relations had become, on those days my parents and I were glad to have each other there. The more people there were to pass the time, the less each of us would have to continually lift in order to keep the weight of the vigil from crushing us. Each time the door to the room opened, each unexpected creak of the hinges, of which there could easily be twelve in an hour — the custodial crew to clean, a technician to test the oxygen valves, nurses and their aides, delivery of the meal tray, a visit from a volunteer — caused a coalescing of the separate energies in the room. From my mother reading the newspaper to Jackie and me working on a jigsaw puzzle. My father asleep in the chair or my brother or sister watching the television. Like the seven fielders behind the pitcher on a baseball team, whose random, disparate wanderings are united into a single, concentrated moment as the ball is pitched, each time the door swung open our heads lifted, the conversation stopped, and the air in the room grew still because it was no longer being breathed. Each false alarm was followed by an awkward intimacy and a few chagrined smiles, with which we hoped to re-create our temporary denial of the news we were girding ourselves for.

So far, each time the pronouncement was made, we had been spared the horror of having to not only imagine, but to confront, our worst fears. This time, when Sheldon Bimberg barreled through the door, five and a half hours after the bone marrow sample had been taken, my parents had already left for home. It was late in the day, heading toward a Friday night. Jackie and I had been alone for the last few hours, and, as Sheldon Bimberg spoke, I had my first glimmer of awareness of the distance that had been steadily developing between my girlfriend and me.

It was not uncommon for me, sometimes three or four times a night, to call Jackie at home for some comfort. If I was scared, or if a fever had cropped up, Jackie was the one I would call. No one else had the level of understanding she did or the degree of compassion that she had been able to show. But, as of recently, Jackie had begun to sound annoyed. She exhibited much less patience for indulging my fears, and I started to get the impression that my calls home from the hospital were being received reluctantly, as if they were an intrusion on the limited amount of time that she had to elude me and my burdensome predicament. My comprehension of this dynamic was vague, however. It only crystallized in my consciousness when the trend was reversed, at least temporarily, by Sheldon Bimberg's proclamation.

"Well, there are no leukemic cells in there," he said, as he burst through the door. That was Dr. Bimberg's style. He blasted into a room spewing forth information, and then stopped himself short, seemingly surprised by whom he'd found inside.

"Oh," he'd say, as if correcting himself, steadying his course. "Hello. Hello." And then he'd gallop on.

"No, no leukemic cells," he said. "But then again it's just as bad. There's nothing there at all. Just empty marrow."

"What does that mean?" I asked.

"Just what it sounds like," I was told. "You've got no counts 'cause there's nothing there. Just fat cells. And there's nothing else we can do for you. We can't take you off the antibiotics because the infection will come back. We can't d.c. the acyclovir because the zoster lesions aren't crusted over yet. So you haven't got leukemia. I mean, that's the good news. But this is really just as bad."

I was speechless. His manner was definitive, extremely energetic. Almost upbeat. It seemed to bear no relation to the information he was imparting. I couldn't think of anything else to ask him, and it seemed he had nothing more planned to say. So he said good-bye.

"Just try to relax, have a good weekend, and we'll check in on you Monday," was what I heard.

It had been some time since I'd gotten the rush of love that comes with a death sentence. This time the emotion hit me more intensely than ever before. I felt like a man who was drowning within sight of shore. I could see each of my dearly beloved friends and family members, but no matter how loudly I screamed, they all continued to laugh and play on the beach. There would be my wife, I imagined. There are my parents and my child. I could just give up, I thought. I could just slip under the water and disappear, and no one would know I had gone. They would never know that I had even been here.

Dr. Bimberg left the room, and Jackie and I sat by ourselves and we cried. We held each other for hours, unable to comprehend what we'd just been told. I knew that a recurrence of leukemia would have meant certain death for me at that point. Hadn't he said this was just as bad? And was that how my life would end, I wondered? With a too loud, too large man telling me there was nothing more that they could do? I hung on to Jackie like I was hanging on to life itself. Not because she could save it for me or change it for me. But because she might be my last taste of it. For the first time in quite a while, she clutched me back. It was the return of the intensity of her emotion that made me first realize that it had gone away. And the only reason I could have it now was because, according to Fred Flintstone, I would soon have to relinquish it forever.

As one of his very wise suggestions, my therapist Yehuda Nir told me that I ought to call the folks at Johns Hopkins. "They are the ones who most recently treated you," he indicated. "Give them a call and see what they have to say." I put in a call, and within an hour, one of the attending physicians had phoned me back.

I told the story of my most recent admission. I described the plummeting blood counts, and the empty bone marrow aspirate. I told the doctor from Baltimore, with as much composure as I could muster, about Dr. Bimberg's assessment that there was "nothing else we can do."

In very calm tones and with reassuring language I was told that what was happening to me was to be expected. "Your blood counts have dropped because of the medications you are on," the doctor said. "We have seen this happen many times. When you are removed from the drugs, your counts will come back up. It may take a long time. But we have never seen a graft that has taken go away."

And after the reassurance came the encouragement. "You hang in there. This might take a while. But don't give up now."

On Monday Dr. Bimberg arrived in my room with a team of doctors visiting from Israel. I asked if I could speak to him privately for a few minutes. When we were alone I told him about my conversation with the doctor at Johns Hopkins. I told him I thought he had done a reckless thing by leaving me with his callous declaration on a Friday evening, with no way to contact him for further information until the beginning of the next week. I told him that he had made me believe that my life was over, and that it seemed, now, that not all doctors would have made that same determination.

Dr. Bimberg offered an apology — of sorts. "If they've never seen a patient lose a graft, I'm happy for them," he said. "But I don't see how they can tell you what's going on from two hundred miles away. I'm the one who's looking through the microscope, and I just told you what I saw. Hey, I didn't know you'd be so concerned. I wasn't concerned. If I upset you, I'm sorry."

My blood counts, as soon as the medications were discontinued, rose steadily and rapidly. The moment I was well enough to leave the hospital I called the doctors at Johns Hopkins again, and I begged them to let me return and complete my outpatient care there. I tried to communicate to them the savage indifference I was encountering in and around New York. There seemed to be an insistence at Sloan-Kettering, I told them, on the validity of a series of equations that held that, if an individual's needs exceed what the institution can comfortably provide, then that individual's needs must therefore be excessive; that whatever level of care the institution is capable of must be adequate, and, therefore, if that care is not good enough, then the patient is unsalvageable. The medical professionals I was dealing with seemed overly inured to the premature deaths of young people, I said, and I was afraid for my well-being in such an atmosphere. After struggling so long to preserve my life I was loath to watch it float out of my grasp while surrounded by people who figured my death was to be expected anyway.

I was told that it was their experience that both the Westchester County Medical Center and Sloan-Kettering provided capable care, and my request was refused. I couldn't really fault them for denying me access; I understood Johns Hopkins's need to preserve the conditions that allowed it to give me such fine care for a time. But it troubled me deeply that they felt the need to cast aspersions on my observations, my experiences, in New York. I had, and I still have, no hidden motive for denigrating any particular facility. But I did think it was important, in the interest of sparing others the dangers I'd faced, that there be a climate in which criticism could be freely expressed, and, when it was, that the criticism be seriously considered. The pressure to improve, I reasoned, could only come from peer institutions, and from their willingness or refusal to refer cases. That way there would be no doubt as to whose care is truly "adequate," because there would be no business for those whose care is not.

Life and love back at home didn't quite live up to the overwhelming flood of intimacy that had followed the most recent pronouncement of doom. The aftermath of a postponed execution is, I imagine, closely related to the mortification felt by passengers after riding in a plane that almost crashes. I don't know if the reports I've heard are true; of terrified passengers reverting to beastly yelps and howls in the face of imminent death. But I can imagine a planeload of traumatized travelers, heading into the safety of the terminal after their near miss, all timorously avoiding the eyes of the strangers who witnessed their regression. Most fearsome, I suspect, would be facing up to one's own, familiar companion, who may have heard and may remember all the frantic yearnings and confessions hurled in the moments of panic. I am familiar with the emotional retreat that can follow an episode of revealing too much; of promising more than can be delivered; of pledging a love too large. When Jackie and I found ourselves spared the brutality of a separation imposed by premature death, what we discovered in its stead was the shame of realizing we meant many of the things we'd said only within a context in which they were inherently impossible. The embarrassment suffered privately then fermented into a resentment of the person whose presence aroused it. And the prospect of living happily ever after was not enhanced, but made to seem ludicrous.

The toll that the last three and a half years had taken became clearer as I tried to shed them and to reconnect with people who had moved on with their lives while mine had been standing still. While my gratitude toward many of the people who had helped me was profound, that was something that I'd had the chance to communicate, in person, on many occasions. After being discharged, though, I eventually began to spend time with some old friends who had sent a card almost four years ago but who hadn't been heard from since. Or, friends who had been among the most devoted for a while and who had sort of slipped off the train along the way.

I had a lot of anger toward those people. I felt abandoned. Eventually, I became worried that I had scared everyone away. Although not nearly as acute as they had been for the previous few years, some medical problems persisted, troubling me at least as much psychologically as they did physically. When I would see or speak with friends, these were the issues on my mind, and I'd give long, detailed descriptions of my symptoms and complain bitterly about my frustration that recovery was taking so long. It was clear that everyone had a limit, a point at which they, too, would jump ship to save themselves. So far, Jackie had been the only person in whom I had so rarely seen the signs of imminent retreat. When I began to recognize the distant numbness that I'd seen in others creeping into her eyes, I finally fell apart myself.

How could I endure any more losses? I thought. My life was still held together by nothing more than my own refusal to surrender it. I was still months from being able to resume anything close to a normal life. I had been warned about some of the bodily functions that would be driven haywire from the ferocious barrage of chemicals that had been run through me, and I was learning to cope with them. The most annoying was also the most common after the treatment protocol I'd received. My sweat glands were temporarily disabled, and for some months, until they switched back on, any exertion resulted in an uncomfortable stinging sensation all over my body. Like a million tiny needles pricking my skin simultaneously. If I wanted to do any exercise I had to be vigilant about regularly wetting myself down with cool water, so as not to overheat my engine and wind up causing damage to the vital parts inside.

In addition to all the more serious repercussions, there was another disturbing problem. My hair hadn't grown back. After each round of chemotherapy prior to the transplant, watching my hair repopulate my head had been an enormous symbol of recovery. Even if I wasn't feeling very well, once the hair had returned, I at least *looked* normal again. As long as I kept my mouth shut about my situation, no one would know that I was any different from them. But since returning from Baltimore, the only action happening up top was that a few wispy colorless hairs grew between the ones that had never fallen out. These continued to get longer and longer until I sported a windswept terrain of patchy, downlike fuzz. If anyone had felt uncomfortable facing me and my illness before, now, without a head of real hair to conceal the evidence of where I'd been, there was no hope of alleviating their anxiety. With Jackie fading away from me emotionally, the question became, What will happen when the strain becomes so great that anyone who can escape must, and will, leaving only me? Trapped, with no way to ease the relentless pressure of the past or to avoid the horrendous uncertainty of the future. Not at all. Not for one second.

All of my planned or projected medical treatments had been completed, except for one. The protocol from Johns Hopkins for post-transplant care called for a series of spinal injections, to be given as soon as a safe level of platelets had been attained. These injections, of a chemotherapy agent called methotrexate, were to guard against the proliferation of any leukemia cells that might have crossed the cerebellum/blood barrier and taken up residence in the brain or in the cerebral-spinal fluid. If it sounds horrible, it is.

Since the administration of the drug required a spinal tap, which until this point had only been the title of a movie I had wanted to see, the procedure required that my platelet level be adequate to avoid any hemorrhaging. But, since my platelet count had never fully rebounded after the transplant, this aspect of the treatment had been long delayed. The likelihood of abnormal cells in my brain was extremely low, it was reasoned; my platelets were sufficient for most activities and might never go any higher. Go about your business, I was told, and we will reassess the situation if ever your platelets come back up. Although it happened with so little fanfare that it was difficult to comprehend, the time had come to begin living the rest of my life.

I had been in touch, intermittently, with my agents for some time already. I had been turning down audition appointments for months, preferring to hold off on my professional reemergence until I was absolutely sure of my durability. But now that the treatments had

been deemed complete, or maybe because The New York Shakespeare Festival's Public Theater was only two blocks from my apartment, I agreed to audition for a production of Shakespeare's *The Winter's Tale*. The hair issue probably also had something to do with it. Most of the calls from my agent had been for films that had roles for college students. This was the height of the "Brat Pack" days, when it seemed that every American film was about people under the age of twenty-five. *Taps*, the movie I had done with Sean Penn, Tim Hutton, and Tom Cruise a few years before the illness, had been one of the first of this era. As every newspaper and magazine published stories about the hottest young actors, I was asked repeatedly by one friend, who knew the story of the last three years of my life and still gave no indication that he was being anything other than sincerely curious, "Why aren't you in the Brat Pack, Evan?"

Even if the years lost to illness had little to do with my exclusion from that club, the fact that I had been rendered hairless was not going to make membership any easier to procure. Although wigs could easily have been used had a director wanted to cast me in a film, I had not yet taken the step of gathering my own private collection of them. I was embarrassed to show up at an audition for clean-cut fraternity characters looking the way I did. But when I read *The Winter's Tale*, I was able to imagine myself playing the part of the Clown, a rustic country fool, without any problems. I went to the audition, feeling a bit self-conscious about suddenly emerging after such a long disappearance, and, after two readings, I was cast in the part from my very first audition back. I was elated by my good fortune and stunned by the ease with which the theater community welcomed me back. And I was amazed to discover that in my life, the most secure thing that existed was an acting career. Two weeks into rehearsals for *The Winter's Tale*, like the statue at the end of the fifth act of the play, my platelets came back to life. I was strongly urged to have the final injections. I had to leave the show.

If anything, short of a recurrence of leukemia or getting hit by a bus, could have crushed my spirit more, I didn't know what it might have been. The one thing I had wanted to be absolutely certain about was that once I took a role, once I proclaimed myself ready and able to perform, I would never again leave a job for any reason having to do with health. I may have established the continued presence of my desirability by getting the first part I tried out for, but now, I was afraid, all people would remember was that Evan Handler was still too sick to work.

Even if I had made my return to the stage a few moments too soon, that didn't keep me out of the view of audiences for very long. Jackie's play, called *Lost and Found,* was being presented in several venues all around New York. Although I was represented as one of the characters in the play, I had been absolutely forbidden from taking part in any of the productions myself. I was asked for advice about who might best portray me, and I received detailed reports about how the various actors were faring as they rehearsed. After this play, Jackie wrote another, called *AML,* for acute myelogenous leukemia. This play was a masterfully written interwoven series of monologues for five actresses, each portraying the same woman at a different stage of caring for her sick lover. In this play, at least, I was given credit for my recovery, and didn't end up dead.

Meanwhile, over at Naked Angels, a theater company formed by many of the friends who had been my regular visitors over the past few years, a one-act festival was being presented. One of these plays, written by Jon Robin Baitz, was the first act of what would later become his brilliant full-length, *The Substance of Fire.* I sat enraptured by the tightening web that my friend Robbie, as I had always known him, was spinning for his characters. About two-thirds of the way through the play, one of the characters delivered a long monologue about his chemotherapy treatment. I listened, astonished, as he expressed to his family onstage many of the same thoughts of life that I had shared with Robbie during his many visits to my bedside.

Those evenings in the theater left me with two different, but equally powerful, impressions. First, I was proud. I was proud to have lived a life that inspired others. I got a sense that, if I had been forced to endure the trials I had, at least they'd affected others to the point where they felt the need to publicly express what they had learned. I have always been obsessive in my desire to be the center of everyone's attention, and the fear of dying had, at least partly, been a fear of being forgotten. My friends' plays were proof that, even in my absence, I had stayed on their minds.

But I also felt trapped. Bound in an indentured servitude to a destiny that I wanted more than anything to reject. As I made the rounds of the theaters in New York, as I appeared in the same places, with the same people as I had for years, everything I could see outside myself looked just the same. It was as if I had been uprooted and given a transplant of fate, rather than of bone marrow. Watching the way my life, the life that I would now be forced to live if I wanted any life at all, had been masticated and incorporated into the creative digestive systems of my friends, left me feeling as if I had become The Subject, fated to live the life out of which others would make art. It started to dawn on me that the living of my life had been my artistic expression for years already, and that perhaps I was doomed and blessed to have become one of those people whose mere existence makes a greater statement than anything they might ever do with it.

*   *   *

I was brought up, in my family, to believe that birthdays are important. And I do. Birthdays tell us things. They are the days that we celebrate a person's life, and they act as markers in time. Between what has been, and what is now. Between now, and what is hoped for someday soon. In my family, we had no Christmas, no reli-

242

gious holidays at all, but we had birthdays. After all that I had been through over the last few years, birthdays had only grown in significance.

My twenty-ninth birthday was the first birthday that fell after the one-year anniversary of my bone marrow transplant. The first birthday since I could consider myself to be *cured* of the disease that had consumed almost five years of my life. But, on my twenty-ninth birthday, it was clear that if Jackie did have any more love to share with me, she no longer had the strength to show it. After working so hard to nurse me, to drag me, back to safety, it had become as if saying "good morning" was just one more thing that Jackie had to do for me.

On my twenty-ninth birthday, Jackie showed no excitement over our accomplishment, and there was no celebration. I told her that it felt like she didn't even give a damn that I hadn't died after all.

Jackie said, "Yeah. That must not feel very good."

And that was the end of that.

I left the house that night reeling and disoriented, feeling cut loose from the only anchor, the only stability, I had known for the last five years. I went to meet my friend Daniel, whose soothing voice had calmed me in some of my darkest moments, to play pool with him and his friend at a billiards hall in Chelsea. I met up with them first at Sam Chinita, an aluminium-sided railroad car diner that serves the ever-puzzling and popular combination of Cuban/Chinese cuisine. I slid into the vinyl booth next to Daniel, and, with the fluorescent lights burning my swollen, bloodshot eyes, I faced his friend Matthew, a total stranger to me, as I tried not to burst into tears. I didn't know what Matthew might have known about me or my history, how much he had been told or what he might have heard. I had called Daniel only a couple of hours earlier, telling him that Jackie and I had broken up and that I was upset.

"Happy birthday," Matthew said, and he pushed something toward me across the Formica table top. "It's a present."

I looked over at the stranger, a smiling, friendly presence, and then down to the gift sitting in front of me. It was a tiny cactus plant, no more than two inches tall. The plant was a single plump stalk, growing out of the sand in a minuscule terra-cotta pot wrapped in green decorative metal foil.

"You can take care of each other," Matthew said. And then we went and played pool.

I took the tiny cactus home with me. The home where I had fought for my life, and loved and lived with the woman who was now gone. I put the cactus on the windowsill where I liked to sit, and I cared for it with intense concentration. I spoke to the cactus, encouraging it to grow and feeding it water and love with all the tenderness that I would have wanted from someone for myself. After about two weeks, I accidentally bumped its baby-sized planter and the cactus fell over onto its side. As I carefully picked it up to plant it back into the soil, I saw that the cactus had no roots at all. In fact, as I examined it, I saw that the cactus was not alive, nor had it probably been from the moment it was given to me. I had been caring for and nourishing a life that didn't exist. I laughed as I tossed the dead cactus into the trash, thinking that Daniel's friend Matthew had given me a gift more perfect than he knew. A dead cactus, supported by nothing but sand. The perfect metaphor, I thought, for the futile efforts Jackie and I had made, for years, to reawaken our corpsified relationship, obviously dead to anyone who looked closely enough, but propped up to give it the illusion of life.

Having lost everything that I had ever had: my hair, my youth, my love, my confidence, my career — everything except my life, which now appeared to be the only thing that was safe — I set about the reconstruction. I'll develop new confidence, I decided. I'll build a new career. I'll embrace adulthood.

That left hair and Jackie. The two things I'd have to learn to live without.

READY OR NOT . . .

As often happens, my reasons for pursuing an acting career had long taken a backseat to my desire to simply *have* a career. As a teenage acting student, I had scoured the underside of Manhattan, studying the bizzarre characters around me, and I tried to re-create them in my classes. My mission in life, I told myself, was to show people the truths they'd rather not confront.

Eventually, however, in the hunt for employment and career advancement, those ideals were largely abandoned. I was tremendously proud of my accomplishments as an entertainer in film and theater. But I had also learned how painfully rare it could be to work on a project that held any deep meaning, any personal connection, for me as a storyteller. The work that I found, while often exciting and provocative, was largely in a mainstream arena, where hard "truths" weren't necessarily what sold tickets. Just as well, I told myself. I'd rather make a living in the mainstream than have only "truth" for dinner each night.

But, while lying in my bed in various hospitals, having felt the full impact of life's force, the old inspiration had crept back in and taken hold. I ached to be back on the stage. The wild swings of the last several years had filled me with an overflow of emotions I felt a consuming need to express. And not only was my desire recharged, but I felt a power, a justification for my presence on that stage, that I'd never had before.

When I envisioned myself back in front of an audience, I saw myself driven by the same urgency I'd felt as a student ten years earlier. I imagined myself giving searing performances, filled with a sadness, rage, and passion for living never before displayed. After all I'd been through, I thought, I would be able to focus an intensity onstage and in front of the camera that would make people want to look away — and not be able to. As usual, I had set my standards rather high.

Six Degrees of Separation, John Guare's smash hit play about the emotional hunger of wealthy, modern-day New Yorkers, produced by Lincoln Center Theater, was my big comeback. While I had been working on various workshops and projects for the past six months or so, some as exciting as an early production of Tony Kushner's masterpiece *Angels in America, Six Degrees* was my first appearance in a major production in more than a year and a half. Except for my brief, interrupted run in *Broadway Bound,* my last appearance on a New York stage was nearly three years past. It had been a frustrating period, as I tried to reestablish myself as a dependable, desirable presence in the eyes of casting directors and producers. I had given several auditions over the course of the six months prior to being cast in *Six Degrees* that I thought would have been, before the illness, more than good enough to secure a role for myself. I could rarely be certain if my medical history was being held against me when I went up for a part, but I could understand it if it was.

I didn't, at the time, consider it to be "discrimination" if someone felt banking on me was a greater risk than necessary in an already perilous venture. But in certain specific instances, such as when I auditioned to play one of the roles in a hit off-Broadway comedy called *Enter Laughing,* and the director apologized to me for being unable to cast me due to the producers' concerns about my health, I would be hurt and angry. Besides feeling upset about the obvious ignorance of the medical facts, I felt cut out of the competition, with no method available to make up the distance I'd fallen behind in the race I experienced my career as being.

As I tried to reclaim my status in the theater- and film-world hierarchy, the difficulty I had accepting my somewhat diminished position was probably mirrored by the people who had replaced me. I went to an audition while I was in *Six Degrees of Separation.* As I sat in the waiting room among the nervous and hopeful actors, my attention was drawn to two young blond men conversing animatedly. One of the men in particular seemed very familiar to me, and I had to resist the temptation to interrupt their chat. First, I thought I might actually know the guy only from seeing him on TV or in the movies — a situation that I've had happen before, and it's embarrassing. Second, whoever he was, even if he did know me, he hadn't seen me in years. And I was wearing a wig. The bone marrow transplant, I'd since learned, had permanently damaged the hair follicles in my head, and so I was wearing a wig for the audition. And when I wear my wig, no one who knows me recognizes me. I'm invisible. Even to some of my most intimate friends and lovers.

It wasn't always that way. When I first began to reenter life after having disappeared six months earlier to go to Baltimore for my bone marrow transplant, the opposite was true. I started popping up at all the places that I used to haunt in the innocent years, seeing all the people who were, at least on some level, my friends. Maybe colleagues is a better word. Friends, colleagues, cohorts, acquaintances. All those people. I'd show up, look around the room, and smile at all the familiar faces, eagerly awaiting the rousing hero's welcome I had imagined so many times during so many dark days. But no one would return my gaze. If I was able to lock eyes with anyone, I got that vague, polite half-smile reserved for strangers who insist on being given some sign that their presence has been noted. And then I realized. No one knew who I was. But, in those days, I was invisible because I was bald. The last time anyone had seen me, I had a head of thick, curly hair.

Thus began an incredibly awkward and painful quest to reintroduce myself to everyone I'd ever known. I went to see a play in which there was a man with whom I'd worked a year or two before, and afterward I stood in a circle of seven or so people that included my friend Donald, the playwright, and his wife, Lynn. I congratulated the actor once, and then a second time, after which he responded, "I'm sorry, do I know you?"

A hushed silence came over the group, broken by my voice. "Yeah, Larry, it's Evan Handler. We worked together in The Young Playwrights Festival last year." He looked utterly confused. Eventually, he gathered himself up and said, "Oh, I'm sorry. I didn't recognize you." Well, no wonder. Not only had I lost my hair, but I had lost ten pounds, and the shape of my face had actually gotten puffier, less angular. A development that has lasted through to today.

And that became routine. Whenever it became necessary to reacquaint someone with me, I'd try to put on an unflustered, ironclad expression and hide whatever mortification I felt in order to spare the poor soul opposite me any hint that my feelings were hurt or that I might have any feelings about anything at all anyway. I myself have still not gotten used to the way I look now. To me, my baldness is an aberration. A cruel joke of the spirits that rule, much as Rip Van Winkle must have felt when he passed a mirror and saw that after a short nap, he had awakened an old man.

I first realized that everyone else had come to accept my new look when I went out with a wig. The same exact syndrome was to be played out, but in reverse. Not only with those who'd met me and gotten to know me since the illness, but also with those who'd been my friends for years and years; they all looked right past me when I showed up with hair, looking just like I used to look. Back when life seemed to make some sense.

So, at the audition, as I studied the blond actor sitting across the room from me, for the first thirty minutes or so I didn't say hello. I didn't call out to him. I didn't even try to make eye contact. I passed on by, pretending that I was a stranger in my own town. Or perhaps a ghost, roaming among those with whom he once lived. Seeing, but unseen.

"Were you in *Biloxi Blues?*"

It was my voice, and one of the blond actors swung his head in my direction. I wondered if it had been a mistake to speak. To engage. The young man's eyes looked at me quizzically and then widened into an expression of utter shock and confusion. He stammered, he sputtered. "Y-y-you. You were very ill!"

He said it again. "You were *very* ill."

"Yes, I was."

"It was . . . I heard. Very serious. Very bleak. I was told."

"Yes. Yes, it was. There was a time when it was."

"I called later, some months. I spoke. It was still very bad. *It was very bad!*"

He seemed to be defending himself. Trying to convince me. I was giving him no argument. I just looked at him with understanding and nodded my head. I knew what he wanted to say, and I was hoping that I could make him feel safe enough to say it.

"I . . . I . . . I thought you were dead!"

What so many had thought, someone finally said. It was so refreshing. Then I thought, Uh-oh. Now I'm going to have to help him get over his horror at what has just come out of his mouth.

"Well, I'm fine now. Cured in fact. Completely healthy."

"Th-th-that's good news. That's very good news."

"Yeah," I said. "Yeah, it really is."

Eventually I started to develop a pride in my new look and all the repercussions of it. I'd had my first wig made with the intention of wearing it everywhere. I was going to be a Mike Nichols kind of guy. Everyone would know I wore a wig, but I would never be seen without it, and people would always wonder if the rumor was true or just some strange showbiz legend. Showbiz legend. Showbiz legend. I was going to be a showbiz legend. But I realized that wasn't for me and I endured the awkwardness and tried to cultivate a new self-image. One of the tattooed survivor. Forever branded by his battles, but refusing to cover his scars for the comfort of anyone else. Sometimes other actors would even express jealousy, as if I had an unfair advantage in being able to alter my looks so completely from day to day. None of them ever shaved their head, though.

At night, I'm still plagued by dreams in which I look in the mirror and see that my hair is growing back. I remind myself of how many times I have been fooled by these dreams before, and, after checking and testing thoroughly, despite my suspicions, I become convinced that I really am awake and that my hair is, indeed, coming back in, as thick and luxurious as it used to be. Then I wake up, confounded by how, or why, I'm capable of playing such a cruel hoax on myself over and over again.

*   *   *

On Saturday morning, May 4, 1991, I was woken up by my phone ringing a bit earlier than it usually does. I stumbled out of bed and into the next room to answer it, and I found my father on the line.

"Hey, buddy," he said. "Are you all right?"

"Yeah, I'm all right," I told him. "What are you talking about? Why wouldn't I be all right?"

There was a short pause. More like a hesitation. "Well," my father said. "Have you seen the papers?"

I hadn't. But I didn't usually run out to buy the newspaper before nine-thirty on a Saturday morning.

"Well, buddy," my father was saying. "Big article in the *Times*. You might want to take a look."

I left my apartment quickly at nine-forty-five and headed to the Gem Spa, the newsstand at the corner of Second Avenue and St. Mark's Place. It's a particularly seedy corner, bustling with activity all night long, that seems to quiet down only shortly before dawn for a couple of hours. The corner, and its strange flow of transient inhabitants, seemed to be reviving itself after its brief respite. I picked up a copy of the *New York Times,* pushed my dollar bill through the Plexiglas window, and stood waiting for my change.

The *New York Times* is, for me, *almost* the perfect newspaper. Reading it each day, for an hour or more, is often the only relief I get from my furious obsessions and self-examination. I hear a lot of people say that they can't stand to read newspapers or watch the TV news because it's too depressing. They'd rather be oblivious to the nightmares in play around them. For me, it's the only way to relax. Reading about horrors that are happening far away — to people other than myself — is the only thing that stops me from thinking about my own problems. It's not that it makes me feel *better* to hear about other people's grief. I'm not *comparing* myself to them; it's just that those stories *take the place* of thoughts that I would have been having if I wasn't reading the paper. And so it feels like a rest. A rather violent, ugly, depressing vacation from myself.

But the *New York Times* doesn't have horoscopes. And, it's pretty short on sexual titillation. That's why, occasionally, I can be spotted peeking at the *New York Post*. I never actually buy the *Post*. I'll look through it if I find it lying around somewhere. But most often I just glance at the headlines when I'm standing around the Gem Spa, waiting for my change from the dollar I've paid to get my dependable, my defendable, my presentable *New York Times*.

When I looked down to where the *New York Post* was piled, I caught only the first word of the day's banner headline. But it was unusual enough to catch my eye right away. "BROADWAY . . . ," it said. Hey, I thought. That's cool, I work on Broadway. I wonder what happened. I wonder if it's about anyone I know. When the whole picture came into focus, I had a sensation that I'm not sure I can describe accurately. The closest I can get is that it felt like I was walking down the street, when I suddenly saw myself go by. It was a "No, wait a minute, that's not right. That can't happen," kind of feeling. On Saturday morning, May 4, 1991, when I stood at the Gem Spa looking down at the cover of the *New York Post,* under the headline "BROADWAY SWORDPLAY TURNS REAL," I saw a picture of myself staring back.

My first impulse was to hide. I had a completely instinctive urge to dive behind something, like a crate, and seek cover. I stopped myself from doing it, but before I could, I did do an amazing thing. I looked all around, very slowly, so as not to draw attention, to see if anyone was watching me. I can only guess that those are both learned responses to hundreds, no, thousands, of movies and television shows that portray fugitives' reactions when they see themselves plastered on the front pages of all the newspapers. Even though I hadn't committed any crime, the fact that my face was on the cover of the *New York Post* made me feel like I must have pushed someone in front of a subway train. Once I was sure that no one was on my trail, of course, I did the next thing that all movie outlaws do. I bought copies of all the papers. I turned my collar up as high as it would go, I drooped my head down low and, looking like the most suspicious character on the corner of Second Avenue and St. Mark's Place, I slunk back home to hide out.

When I walked through my front door, the clock read nine-fifty-eight. I'd been gone for thirteen minutes. The phone was ringing, and there were nine messages waiting on the answering machine.

When I picked up the receiver to answer the call, before I could utter the word "hello," before I heard the sound of another human being on the line, I heard the beep that told me another call was waiting. I got the feeling that my location had been compromised.

I had conversations with three people on the phone that morning. During each of those calls, I got three more on call waiting. I couldn't hang up the phone without hanging up on someone. Although I had spent my entire life fantasizing about fame, now that I was getting a tiny taste of it, all I wanted was to find someplace where no one knew who I was. After about an hour of complete madness I fled my apartment, with the phone ringing, deciding that the best place to be anonymous in New York was at a major sporting event. I got on the number six train for Grand Central, then transferred to the number seven to Queens, where I knew the New York Mets had a game that day against the Cincinnati Reds. Sitting on the subway, with my picture staring back at me from the cover of dozens of *New York Posts* being read by the other passengers, I felt that surely the world, or else I, had gone mad. I leaned back against the seat, closed my eyes, and made believe I was on the run in an Alfred Hitchcock movie.

Two nights before, in front of about five hundred people at the Walter Kerr Theater on Forty-eighth Street, I had quit my job. I was doing a play on Broadway called *I Hate Hamlet,* costarring with a somewhat well known, tall, brooding Scottish actor. In the theater there is an ancient tradition of superstition. One of the more fearsome rules to break is the utterance anywhere inside a theater, for any reason, of the title of William Shakespeare's play *Macbeth.* Should the dreaded word be spoken, there are theater professionals who will react as if their lives have been threatened. They will scream, their faces distorted by a mixture of rage and fear, until the transgressor performs one of the bizarre rituals that supposedly breaks the spell.

I have seen dignified elderly actors shove their colleagues out of a dressing room, refusing them readmittance until they have spit on the ground and spun themselves around three times.

Some theater professionals refuse to speak the word anywhere at all. Several productions of that particular play are said to have been cursed, and the curse is passed along to other productions whenever the title of "The Scottish Play," as it's cautiously referred to, is carelessly bandied about. During the four weeks of rehearsals and the six weeks we had been running *I Hate Hamlet,* the behavior of The Scottish Actor (as I had just as superstitiously taken to calling him) had been, in the genteel, lawsuit-shy language of the press, "unpredictable." When, after ten weeks of witnessing remarkable amounts of early-afternoon alcohol consumption, every conceivable tantrum, every imaginable fit of fear-induced bullying, after enduring every possible glare and growl of vituperation, The Scottish Actor began berating me in mid-performance, I felt close to my breaking point. About twenty minutes later, during the first act's climactic sword fight, when he wound up and smacked me with a three-foot-long piece of stainless steel, I decided that I'd had enough and left the stage.

I didn't know, in the moments immediately following my departure, if I was mostly angry, or embarrassed, or proud of myself. My reflection in the dressing room mirror was puzzling. I saw fury in my eyes. My face was a mask of rage. I wondered if I had been cowardly in running away, rather than staying and confronting him. But what would I have done? Turned and attacked him? Had a brawl right there on the stage? I pulled down the back of my costume pants and saw a seven-inch-long welt swelling up; a perfect, double-edged, bright red imprint of the blade.

My mind searched for other options. I supposed I could have attempted to calmly finish the act. But surely, enduring a public beating without defending oneself in any way is beyond anyone's responsibilities. I had already complained bitterly for weeks about the lack of enforcement of any safety measures surrounding the sword fight. The Scottish Actor had simply refused to participate in the nightly fight rehearsal required by the actor's union, usually appearing at the theater minutes after the curtain was scheduled to go up. As each of my complaints was brushed aside, other cast members had routinely pulled me aside and urged me to push harder for some action. "It looks dangerous," I was told. "You're going to lose an eye out there."

Yes, I had done the right thing; the only thing I could do, I told myself. At least this way, I reasoned, the bullying blowhard was left holding the bag. At least he would have to deal with the embarrassment of finding himself left alone on stage, with no explanation as to why.

"Well, should I sing?"

It was The Scottish Actor's voice, coming to me over my dressing room monitor. I heard him go on. "It seems an actor who has missed a few parries has become upset and elected to leave the stage. Unless one is very, very sick, this is a terribly unprofessional thing to do. We'll ring down the curtain and begin the second act in a few minutes." He left the stage to a round of applause.

Well, I thought. Touché. I spoke briefly with one of the producers of the show; I told him I wouldn't be back; I left the theater and I went home.

Whenever I've told people any part of the story since then, when I report that I thought nothing more would come of it than five hundred or so people having a good story to tell when they got home that night, I get a lot of indulgent smirks thrown my way — as if no one believes that I could possibly have been so naive. But I left the show on a Thursday night. Nothing had changed dramatically in my life. I just didn't have to go to the theater for my dose of indignities the next night, and I was glad. Certainly the world wasn't paying any more attention to me than it had been the day before. Friday night I went to sleep early. I had gotten only three phone calls that day.

When I got to Shea Stadium I checked my answering machine back home. There were twelve new messages — including calls from CBS News, *Hard Copy,* and the *Daily Telegraph* in London. To me it seemed obvious that no one was really excited about what had happened inside the Walter Kerr Theater on Thursday night. They were all foaming at the mouth over the fact that someone else had printed a story about it before them, on Saturday morning.

The question asked first, by anyone who was at all close to me at the time, was, "Do you think you would have done the same thing before you were sick?" Even those who didn't pose it as a question were making the same assumptions. "How brave," I was told. "How admirable. Saying 'I've been through too much already to put up with this. I have better things to do with my time.'"

I can't dispute the fact that those were my feelings. But I also can't deny that I had been having those feelings for weeks before I was willing to act upon them. I would try to explain to people that I was glad to have, finally, asserted myself. But the stance that would have been admirable, I countered, would have been walking away when there was really something to lose. What I would like to have gained was the courage to refuse to participate in such an unbalanced and abusive power structure from the moment it became apparent, before I had taken my shot at succeeding in spite of it. Ultimately, I seized an opportunity to escape, no more. I was stunned, really, by how little difference there was between my behavior and what might have been in the past. I was proud of what I had done. But the moment of pride had come after many long weeks of disappointing myself.

With all the attention that was heaped upon the *I Hate Hamlet* episode, its legend quickly eclipsed my reputation for any work I might have previously been known for. The incident was reported on internationally for weeks, and then again a full eight months later, as part of the year-end highlight issues of *Time, Newsweek,* and the Sunday *New York Times.* I had become "the guy who walked off the stage." While a bit intoxicated by the notoriety, I was still worried about how this impression might influence potential employers. I was also furious about the humiliation I had suffered, both that night and in the months afterward. As I became embroiled in a union proceeding to receive pay for the full length of my contract, due to management's failure to uphold union regulations and provide a safe work environment, I realized that no one involved with the production was going to volunteer to verify my charges. Although we had all complained and suffered together, apparently there was something about my response, my refusal to toe the company line — however long delayed — that set me apart. For the first time, I was able to pull back and see the events in perspective. I realized that, compared to where I had been in my life, this was a meaningless engagement. The stakes — money, honor, reputation — while seemingly enormous, were really about pride, and had very little to do with one's ability to exist. The distinction I was able to make, at last, was the difference between forces that are annoying and those that pose a real threat. It's not a matter of life and death, I told myself, even though it felt like it was. And, in the painful, but, I'd like to believe, mature act that probably would *not* have happened at any time in my life before, I decided that it was better to cut my losses and find happiness down the line than to stay shackled to an unpleasant experience in a quest for ever elusive justice. I dropped my sword again, and I walked away from another fight.

THE BLUE WARRIOR

A lot has been written, since writing came to be, about what it is like to be ill. Anatole Broyard became intoxicated by his illness. Flannery O'Connor felt she had traveled to another country. I think that anyone who has ever been sick, with even a cold or the flu, knows exactly how it feels. But I would step back, make a half turn, and say that only those for whom illness has at one time been their companion know what it feels like to be well.

Before I had leukemia, I thought "feeling well" was a neutral state. If I had a toothache; if I had a sore throat; if food poisoning was wrenching my intestines and causing me to shiver and sweat, these felt like dazzling intrusions on my natural, restful composition. A flat graph, showing no data at all, broken by temporary spikes of vivid, unpleasant sensation. "Feeling good," I realized, had really been a translation for "feeling nothing."

Only after high fever, nausea, and furious pains wove themselves around every fiber of my neurology; when drooling and vomiting were so accepted that I carried a plastic pea-green basin with me everywhere I went; when physical torment reached its apogee with anal fissures that made a half-centimeter orifice feel like a swollen seven-ton tumor did I begin to comprehend, and cherish, the immeasurable ambrosial delights that caressed my senses in the absence of such interference.

When any of these or any of the other half-billion maladies that made up my illness receded, I would try to distinguish between and catalogue some of the previously ignored sensations of wellness. The simple act of inhaling air effortlessly, as opposed to the labored panting of my sickbed, became a practically orgasmic pleasure. I rediscovered the presence of the sticky-sweet taste of oxygen in the air, even in the cloying polluted haze of midtown Manhattan. This was a taste I hadn't been familiar with since my childhood, and that I'd since forgotten I had ever known. Walking through Central Park, entranced by the spongy crunch of my shoes as they snapped apart decaying twigs and leaves — and enjoying the sensuousness of my shoes rhythmically massaging my sock-covered feet — I took deep, appreciative breaths. I stopped in my tracks when the taste of the air brought back a torrent of memories. I stood rapt in the park, as my mind took me back to the summers I'd spent playing at the lake down the road from my family's house.

"The raft" was the wooden platform that floated just a short distance from the beach and dock. The water out by the raft was probably about ten feet deep. When a Frisbee is released under water, it slowly rises to the top — but it doesn't become visible in a murky lake until it is within two or three feet of the surface. For the game we played, the "hider" would dive down into the blackness of the water, where his or her goal was to fool all the other players by getting them to expect the Frisbee to rise somewhere far from where it ultimately did. You couldn't do this unless you could hold your breath. For a long, long time.

The Buttons were superhuman masters of this. Three brothers, Alan, Richie, and Jamie, all comic book specimens of All American, Eagle Scout athleticism. Older than the rest of us, one of the Button brothers would dive down into the water. First his blond head, and then his perfect, chiseled body would disappear. Moments later, bubbles would be released on the other side of the raft from where we were all lined up. As we dashed over to watch on that side, determined not to be fooled, another burst of bubbles would come up from the side we'd just left. By the time the Button brother resurfaced, minutes later and gasping for air, we would all be scattered over the four sides of the raft, completely bewildered not only as to where the Frisbee was, but also as to how such a feat was even possible. When someone finally located the Frisbee, we were much less impressed by them than we were by the brilliant display by the brother who'd hidden it. That's why it became so urgent to win the race to find it. The finder became the next hider, and when we won the right to take the Frisbee down, we all tried our best to imitate the miracles we had grown used to seeing, and to leave our friends as admiringly astonished as we had felt ourselves.

In Central Park, sitting on a rock, tickling myself by rubbing my fingers over its rough surface, I remembered how the air would taste after I clawed my way back up to the surface of the water, having nearly asphyxiated myself in trying to pull off a Frisbee dive to rival one of the Button brothers'. Just before reemerging, I would feel the burning in my lungs reach a crescendo, and the roaring in my ears while I was still submerged would be replaced by the other kids' screams as I shot out of the water and sucked fresh air into my lungs. After I was deprived of breath for two or three minutes, the taste was distinctly sweet, and it stuck to the very top of the back of my throat. There it would linger until, after a few more breaths, it was taken for granted once again. Then the flavor of the sweetest scent we know faded into the background, as if it had never been there at all — as if it wasn't there in every single breath we take.

*   *   *

Bone marrow transplantation erases the immune system's memory of all it has been exposed to. A twenty-seven-year-old man recovering from the procedure has twenty-seven years of immunity to reacquire. There is no way to speed the task or to condense it into a shorter time span. Like a newborn child, he will be safe enough from most of the serious threats to his system, but vulnerable to a slowly narrowing range of annoying infections. I myself, seven years past my transplant, am considered to have perfectly normal immune function. That is, normal for a seven-year-old child. The cells swimming through my adult body, whose task it is to swarm and attack, are, on a daily basis, being confronted by particularly adult adversaries. Few seven-year-olds kiss with their mouths open. If they come into contact with someone else's sexual secretions, there is something seriously wrong. Alcohol is not a drug of choice for most first- or second-graders, nor do immune-impairing levels of stress feature prominently in their lives, as they do with most adults. And, in direct opposition to most of the grown-ups that I know, when children are tired enough, lo and behold, they lie down and go to sleep. It is in adulthood that we come to sense the limit to the length of a day, or the impending crunch of a deadline hurtling toward us. We try to manipulate time and to squeeze more productivity out of smaller amounts of it. With less energy left in our reserves than in our younger human counterparts, we make demands on our bodies that would lay a seven-year-old child out cold. My seven-year-old child, my second-grade immune system, has had some trouble keeping up.

This fact has provoked in me a preoccupation with the possibility of falling ill, and a fear of situations that might increase the odds. For the first few years posttransplant, when colds always became sinus infections, which were followed by strep throats, I was already exhausted from the reality of these inconveniences. But, even when I was feeling well, my fear over when the next attack would come made enjoying myself a monumental task. An evening out in a smoky bar, packed with the steaming, germ-laden breath of native New Yorkers would only accentuate my chronic sense of dread, my hypervigilance in terms of watching for symptoms, as I'd wait for the inevitable scratchiness on my soft palate; the familiar buildup of pressure as the glands in my neck expanded; the throbbing beat of the headache that started behind the eyes. Gloom and despair would engulf me, mixing with the physical sensations, as I realized my defenses were being overwhelmed yet again, and I was in for another week of aches and pains, of wheezes and sneezes, of fever and lethargy. Another week of waiting for something else, of waiting for relief, of waiting, waiting, waiting; wishing that a part of my life would fade away so I could move on to whatever might come next. Two weeks out of each month, after clawing myself bloody to get it back, I'd be waiting, wasting, wishing my life away.

This aspect of my life has also tested the bounds of love and devotion in my relationships with women since the illness. As a relationship progresses from casual and electric to prolonged and thoughtful, the romantic glow of perfection surrounding all aspects of the other individual wears off — even the romance attached to that enduring legend: the defiant, heroic survivor. While I'm certain that my exploitation of this American myth has attracted many to me, I have been repeatedly crushed as I've witnessed the disappointment of my lovers as they discover me to be someone who has been weakened by the very trials that give me the appearance of strength. As the cost of the legacy is revealed, as the frequent colds cast light on the justifiable but mind-boggling hypochondria, which exposes the environmental paranoia, which illustrates the depressive response to a world in which death is inevitable, I can recognize the second thoughts clicking into their minds like disks being sucked into a computer. People are unprepared for the reality of the toll that's been taken. There has been a point in each of the relationships I've had since Jackie when it became clear that the woman has begun to wonder, What did I get myself into here?

Several relationships have blossomed and broken up since the transplant. In an emotional crisis that includes the loss of love, especially a loss that involves the fear of being abandoned or being left alone, one of the first thoughts to rush into my head is, What if I got sick again now? Who would be there? Who would take care of me? I couldn't possibly have survived without Jackie last time. I barely survived with her. This can't be happening. I'm going to get sick again and die alone. Somehow, the two pains — the loss of love and the loss of life — are intimately related. As if any loss, every loss, would be as devastating as the ultimate loss I've succeeded in avoiding so far.

Then the real perversion will kick in and I'll think, Hey, if I got sick and wound up in the hospital, then she'd come back. Sure. She'd come running. And I wouldn't even tell her what was happening. She'd hear it from someone else and desperately try to find me, and she'd feel incredibly guilty for however she might have wronged me. This thought process takes hold regardless of whether I've been left or the breakup was by mutual consent or if I've done the leaving myself. I'll imagine my ex-lover rushing to sit by my bed and hold my hand, then willing me to get well so we can live together happily and triumphantly, with nothing that can ever come between us or even upset us ever again, because we know the value of life, and we know how precious and fleeting it is, and we'll never ever forget the lessons we've learned.

Then I'll think, *Holy shit, Evan. What are you doing? What the fuck are you thinking?!* Because now I've really scared myself. Now that I've had these thoughts, I become afraid that I will really wind up subconsciously giving myself leukemia again out of some kind of demented self-pitying spite. The same as when my mother made me angry as a kid. I'd destroy my favorite toy right in front of her. To show her how much she had hurt me.

I can understand the difficulty that my situation presents to anyone who doesn't inhabit it themselves. If my life didn't require that I possess knowledge of the kinds of tragedy that can befall someone, I don't think I would choose a companion who introduced that knowledge to me. But for all the noise I may have made at home, for all the whining and parading I do and have done, there is much that I keep to myself.

For a period of years after the transplant, once a month, I would go for a blood test. It is a routine that continues today, although far less often. It is nothing but the most basic of all blood tests, a CBC — complete blood count. A machine counts the number of cells in a certain amount of blood, differentiates between the cell types, and prints the numbers out on a piece of paper. It takes about fifteen minutes to get the results. For the past several years, I have gotten my blood drawn in the outpatient lab of New York University Medical Center. I wait for them to hand me the slip, and I take it up to the office of my doctor. But I don't proceed directly there.

I have no need for the numbers to be interpreted for me; it's the simplest of charts to read. Even if one were not acquainted, as I am, with the normal range of numbers, they are printed right there with the results. Each time I have my blood tested, I wait for the slip of paper to be handed to me, and, feeling like the judge, jury foreman, and defendant all in one, I go off to a quiet corner to read the verdict and learn whether I get to keep living my life. The chances of recurrence are slim. Minuscule. But I fear the worst every time I go.

Occasionally the machine will print out numbers that are alarming. Occasionally, the machine will say something like "abnormal white blood cell population." This is exactly what the machine would say if I were to have leukemia. On those occasions, I have to sit in the waiting room, waiting for the doctor to see me. I sit for an hour, sometimes two, and I imagine saying good-bye to my friends. I imagine myself getting the news of a recurrence and wonder whom I would call first. I watch the doctor come and go, ushering in one patient after another, and I want to scream. *"No! Wait! I have to go now! Take me! I think I'm dying and I have to find out! Help! Save me! Save me! Please, save me! I have to know now!"*

I might have to wait two hours before it is my turn to see the doctor, and another until she can check the slide for herself. Then she'll tell me I'm all right, and sometimes I believe her.

If I share these anxieties with anyone, it's still most likely to be Jackie. She and I are the best of friends now, and we speak all the time. In the midst of our other relationships, our loves and more petty obsessions, we have found a deep need for the other's presence. When I'm dealing with the difficult repercussions of all that once transpired, I get the feeling that Jackie is the only person who truly understands. When we get together, or have long phone conversations from wherever in the world we happen to be, we share our difficulties and depressions, our glimpses of beauty and our occasional ecstasies. We both seem to get a unique comfort from sharing our present-day skirmishes with an old war buddy who fought the big one alongside us.

Another inevitable aspect of our visits, as well as any time I visit with my parents, is reminiscence. There has rarely been a conversation with Jackie in years that hasn't gone back to those days. Often she will be able to recall in great detail events that I have completely forgotten, and I'll roam through her memory, exploring its hidden corners, as my mind gropes to uncover and dust off its own.

A few years ago Jackie took me out to dinner to celebrate my thirtieth birthday. We sat together, across a candlelit table, and we found ourselves roaring, hysterical, as we pored over the most gruesome details of the years of suffering. No one's agony was spared. We laughed, and cried, over the horrors that we'd experienced as well as those that we'd witnessed others going through. Eventually we paused and looked up through our tears, and asked each other, as we always do, why it is that we spend so much time on such a twisted ritual.

I had the distinct feeling, that particular night, that I was at a seance. Here were two old lovers, catapulted out of their youths and away from any protective denial of their own mortality, who would convene every so often to conjure the spirits of the kids that they once knew each other to be. Children, really, whom they had loved and who had loved each other. Children that they had watched die, from across the room, with only the other as witness. There seems to be in each of us a barrier, impenetrable without the other one's presence, between that child and the adult that was fashioned out of its corpse. There was no gradual transition, no lengthy metamorphosis. Only an execution and reincarnation, and so, no traceable path back.

Mixed in with all the sorrow and breast beating, there is also, between us, an astonishing sense of accomplishment. In Jackie's play, the one written in the apartment we shared during the depths of the ordeal, the dead boyfriend, in the scene where he appears to the heroine, asks her, "What's the most important thing you ever did? What are you most proud of in your life?"

"Helping you," she says.

When Jackie and I get together, the absurdities that once provoked such anger now mix with them a sense of triumph, and those triumphs are looked back on with some degree of . . . longing?

Because that was our youth. The last gasp of it. And no matter how painful the passage into adulthood might have been, it still holds the closest ties to a childhood that's missed.

*   *   *

As I began looking through the notebooks I'd kept during the first six months of the medical crisis, I read entry after entry about a man deeply in love with the life he was in fear of losing. A man who swore on his soul that he would never — could never — again be so foolish as to feel anything other than privileged about his existence, regardless of where it took him. "Just give me life," this man had written, on page after page. "Just give me my life back, and I will never need anything more than that again."

Reading those notebooks was a jarring and surreal experience. It was difficult to believe, as I sat hunched over them, in the same rooms of the same apartment where they had been written, that those thoughts had come from me. And yet, I had a clear memory of having written them. And the rereading of those passages reinfused each cell of my body with the physical sensations of terror and desire that had originally inspired me to write them down. So, what had happened between then and now? The idea of my own inability to maintain the lessons learned in the struggle, especially since I had assigned the learning of those lessons as the *reason* for the struggle, was a horrifying concept to confront. I had no explanation for how a man who had once felt the preciousness of life so clearly could lose hold of it so quickly, and I was forced to ask myself the question, If being miraculously rescued from the clutches of an almost always fatal disease wasn't enough to leave a lasting sense of wonder and appreciation, then what hope could there possibly be of my ever gaining lasting contentment?

I began, slowly, to write down some of the war stories. To craft the diaries and memories into some kind of cohesive narrative. I tried to infuse them with the issues they were raising for me as I reexamined them and, eventually, I hoped to collect them into a theatrical piece I might perform. The isolation I felt from others, prompted by the glaringly different experiences we'd had over the past several years, was dissipating terribly slowly. I hoped that sharing with other people where I'd been might help to bridge the chasm that had opened between.

And the writing and performing of the piece, the reimmersion in the memories and the revisiting of the emotions, did have an effect. When I first started telling the story to people, their reactions filled me with feelings of triumph that I had rarely been able to reach on my own. I remembered that one of the goals I had set for myself years before at the Simonton Center in California — one of the purposes I'd assigned to my life that made the effort to save it worthwhile — was to hold myself up as an example, so that others wouldn't have such a hard time imagining their own success. As I began the process of performing the piece regularly in theaters, I got a tremendous sense of exaltation in recounting the determination and commitment that had resulted in my being able to be in the room to speak about it. Dressed ceremonially in the blue linen blazer, blue T-shirt, and blue jeans I'd chosen to compliment the subtle blue-tinged lighting scheme, I felt like the subject rendered in a mesmerizing pastel drawing I'd been given as a gift. *The Blue Warrior* was a depiction of a round, hairless head, done in hues of yellow and blue, whose face was streaked with what looked like war paint. The expression was one of sadness, with a thinly concealed ferocity lingering just beneath. The title was clearly intended to convey both a literal and figurative description of the character portrayed, a duality that I was experiencing in my performances. Each time I stepped in front of the audience to tell my story, I felt like a blue warrior, with a painted face, heading into battle. And it was those battles, that reengagement, that helped me to then walk down the street with the awestruck amazement I'd imagined would inspire every waking minute of the rest of my life. I felt I was floating through a private reunion with all the tiny wonders of the world. I tried to accept as a natural human drive the desire to submerge the painful memories, and so, to submerge the knowledge gained through those experiences as well, and I vowed to always be on guard against it, and to fight my way back whenever I felt myself losing ground.

About an instant after making those vows, a familiar cycle began repeating itself through the few short months of the off-Broadway run of that show. While at first there had been a pure joy in the telling of my story, it wasn't long before those feelings were upstaged by more current demands. Like the ad wasn't big enough; the review wasn't good enough; the audience isn't laughing hard enough.

One particular day, as I trudged my way up the dingy, graffiti-scrawled stairway of the Second Stage Theatre in New York, as I entered the green room backstage — the "Ian McKellan Green Room," as the plaque read — a room that was as fresh and clean as any boiler room I'd ever entered in my life, I was dreading the performance that lay ahead of me. I don't remember if it was the special "Family Day Matinee" or the "Singles Night" that time around, but neither one of them seemed a very good marketing strategy for a bare-stage monologue about one angry man's leukemia. Sitting slumped on the filthy, sagging couch that was kept outside the dressing rooms, I tried to talk myself down from the spinning rage I was working myself into. I reminded myself of some of the promises I'd made years before in various hospitals, in various stages of decay and recovery. There was the time in Johns Hopkins when all I wanted was a cooler. An ice-filled chest to take to the beach and keep filled with cold drinks and fresh fruits. At that time, I hadn't eaten any food in five weeks. The chemotherapy had utterly destroyed the flesh lining my mouth and throat, and, while I was being fed intravenously, due to the indescribable pain, even my saliva had to be spit out rather than swallowed. By the time the tissue healed, my sense of taste had been completely destroyed. I would sit in a state of sad bewilderment as Jackie ate meals in the room. I'd smell the roast chicken, the buttery mashed potatoes.

"How is it, sweetie?" I'd ask. "Taste good?"

"Mmmmmm! Ummm Hmmmm."

I would hold a piece of fruit — a piece of sliced orange, say, or maybe a fresh peach. The smell of the fruit would fill my head, it would fill the whole room. I was fascinated by how intense this aroma was, and I would become convinced that if I could smell it so strongly, I must be able to taste it. I would pop a section of the orange into my mouth, bite down, and wait for the flavor explosion. Then I would weep from frustration as I was left with what felt like a mouthful of wet ash. Not to worry, though. I was assured that the problem "almost always" went away within a few weeks.

This particular horror was happening in the midst of various mind-blowing fevers, and I began to dream, out loud, about what I would do with my life once I had it back. With Jackie in the room I talked on and on about this cooler and what kind of things I'd keep inside. This was not a passing fancy. I became convinced that this was how I was going to spend my days once I was well. This was going to be the focus of my life. Jackie would bring catalogues to the hospital, and I would spend hours fantasizing over the most impressive models; drooling, literally, over the shiny plastic ice chests and the sophisticated features that I could never have dreamed existed.

One day, as I was speaking with the doctors, I idly popped a slice of fresh peach into my mouth, and . . . I thought it was burning up my flesh. An enormous eruption on the right side of my tongue. I could taste the peach. I could taste the peach! I ran to the doorway of my room and shouted to the nurses who had suffered through my suffering with me. "My taste came back! It's coming back! My taste is back!"

I had fallen in love. I fell in love and I swore that every bite of food I ever took from that moment on, every bite of life, would taste as sweet and surprising as that first taste of peach. And that was the beginning of my problem. I had gotten well, and I never went to the beach. I didn't own a cooler. The fact is, even if it's a sad fact, that as circumstances change, as options change, so do desires. When I again came to trust that I would have the next five days, the next five months, the expectations grew. Grew even greater than the expectation that every moment should feel just as miraculous as that first taste of peach. The trick, I told myself, would be to learn to relish the mundane, to have an excited involvement with it, in spite of my disappointment that anything could ever become mundane again.

I pulled myself up off the couch, determined to give the Second Stage subscribers the best goddamned singles night they'd ever seen. I passed into the long, skinny dressing room and turned toward my chair — the one farthest on the right, with sixteen empty ones to my left — and I noticed a large gift-wrapped package sitting on the counter in front of the mirror. Opening night had come and gone, so the sight was unexpected, and the package was a mystery. I opened the card that was attached, and I saw that it was from Jackie. "Congratulations," she had written. "Happy Springtime."

I reached down and started to tear the paper off. As I peeled through the layers of wrapping, I saw that it was some kind of a handle that caused the odd shape. Narrower at the bottom than at the top, and tenting up in the middle. And then I gasped. As I saw enough of the gift revealed I made a sound that I'd never heard come out of myself before. Because it was a cooler. A miniature, red-and-white, hard-plastic Rubbermaid cooler, just big enough for a six-pack.

I stood still for a long time, with my hand clamped tight over my mouth. When I had calmed down enough, I reached for the cooler so I could move it to another table. I was already late in getting ready for the show, and I figured I'd give myself a chance to get as emotional as I needed to after it was done. But, when the cooler was much heavier than I expected it to be, I realized that there had to be something inside. I snapped the handle down from the top to release the lid, and the smell hit me hard, like a fist in my face. I pulled the red cover aside, and I saw that the cooler was filled with peaches.

*　　*　　*

While the love, admiration, and appreciation I feel for my family now doesn't diminish the memory of the anger and disappointment I felt then, neither does that anger or disappointment in any way diminish my awareness now of how much my family sacrificed for me. My feelings are difficult to reconcile. I owe my parents my life — twice over. They responded to a crisis with every ounce of energy in their souls, and better than most people ever could have. My survival is no less their victory than my own. In spite of that, at the time, I still expected more. It undoubtedly says much more about me than it does about them or their abilities. My perceptions tend to run toward the recognition of what is wrong, and the impulse to make it right. It is that level of demand and expectation that helped me to survive.

I think often now about my parents and what they must have gone through as a result of my illness. What they must have been steeling themselves for. I've spoken with them about it since, and my father has told me, "I had to protect myself. I had to pull away. If you had died . . . I couldn't allow myself to go down with you. I had to think about the rest of the family, about keeping us together."

When I hear a comment like that, it shows me that the pragmatism I brought to my fight was no accident. It's clear where it came from. And I'm grateful that he passed it on.

The doctors and nurses and hospital staff, my parents and siblings and friends — it is not only these others by whom I've felt let down. For my chronic discontent I blame no one but myself. I cannot satisfy myself any more than others have satisfied me in the past. I am a man impossible to please. It's what got me through. And it's what keeps me from finding contentment here on the other side. While I try to continually remind myself to live each day as if it might be my last one, the knowledge that every day could be my last usually makes me too sad to enjoy them.

When I get a call on the phone, as I often do, asking my advice or assistance for someone confronting an unthinkable diagnosis, I tend to have a knee-jerk reaction that would have sent me into a blind fury when I was ill. I almost inevitably think, Oh, Jesus. The poor bastard hasn't got a chance. I have to stop myself, and try to remember what I've learned. I have to remind myself of what I've proven to the world. The fact that I've been among the first to lose sight of my own example baffles me still.

My friend Lisa called me recently. I'd known since we met less than two years before that she was "dealing with" cancer. She told me as soon as I was introduced to her. "So it's in remission?" I'd asked her then.

"No, no," she said. "I'm *dealing* with it." Some months into our friendship, looking back on that day, she told me, "You should have seen your face. Your eyes turned into little toy guards." I decided then that I was going to try to open my heart to Lisa, to push through whatever it was that made me want to hide from anyone facing similar obstacles to those I had faced.

On the phone Lisa sounded sad and frightened. She rarely shared her medical trials with me, and when she did it was usually with an upbeat sardonicism. Today, though, there were tears in her voice. And fatigue.

"Oh, I saw my doctor this morning," she said. "It was eleven-thirty and he asked me to come back at three. I looked at him and said, 'Okay. Why don't you just tell me now?' He told me he wanted his partner to be there with him." My friend Lisa, thirty-four years old and riddled with cancer, had already lost her vision in one eye, and suffered from nerve damage that severely limited the use of her left hand.

"I already know what they're going to say, Evan," she went on. "But I don't want them to amputate my left hand. I know the cancer is in my wrist, but I'm extremely attached to that hand. And I want to stay attached to it."

I just thought, How am I supposed to leave the house and relate to anyone after hearing something like that? And I've got no excuse, I thought. No excuse for wasting away the time I never should have had to begin with.

Later, Lisa had her suspicions confirmed. "They told me the cancer was spreading at an alarming rate. They feel the best treatment would be to amputate my left arm just below the elbow. I told them no."

After a pause she went on. "So I've been told, unless one of the experimental treatments works or the cancer stops of its own volition, that the time frame for everything will be much shorter than what I was originally told."

We spoke about her decision, and I tried my best to be helpful. But I felt as lost and inept as I'd found my visitors years before. I had no idea how to face my friend who was so stoically facing her own death. The fact is, I never confronted death as anything more than a terrifying specter that I always managed to push away. If anything, my experiences have left me with an even stronger *denial* of death than ever before. I know the fear of it well. But as for acceptance, I never got close.

A lot of young people I've known have died since I was first ill. At least a dozen in ten years, the oldest of them not much over forty. Jeff Lowenthal; Kevin Gheen; A. J. Antoon; Greg Handler; Rema Hort; Jonathan Alper; Martin Herzer; Linda Spoor; Ralph Marrero; Andy Louie. And, yes, I'm sorry to say, Willie Dingle. Though I didn't learn of it until seven years later, Willie Dingle died on March 13, 1988 — less than two months after I saw him looking so well. Willie was twenty-three years old.

Where did these people go, to where did they disappear? I've heard about the concept of "survivor's guilt," and I've always kept alert for the pangs of it. I've definitely felt embarrassed in the presence of an obviously doomed companion, and I have felt like hiding from the parents of deceased friends or acquaintances. Because of the relationships that were forged during my horrible years, it's always seemed an odd reversal of fortunes to confront someone else's grief over an early death that I'd thought was meant for me. But mostly I walk away from such encounters feeling lucky. Shaken; frightened for my own future in this treacherous world; and glad it wasn't me. I classify myself as one of the very luckiest of the unluckiest people to have ever lived.

As the years pass, so with them does much of my immediate terror. But it is always accessible, and rather than feeling that it has dissipated, it seems more to have gone slightly dormant. In the days leading up to and stretching through the illness I became convinced that illuminated street lamps would switch themselves off whenever I passed underneath. This was a phenomenon that had first started occurring, or that I had first noticed, shortly before I met Jackie. On my very first date with her I mentioned it, only to have, in the middle of the next sentence, a streetlight go dark as we walked beneath. I came to believe, after the diagnosis about a year later, that this was a manifestation of some kind of anti-life force. Each time it would happen I was filled with dread, certain that it was a sign that there was still some terrible spiritual imbalance that was affecting the electrical currents around me. It still happens every so often, and I've got to drive it out of my mind immediately or else I will obsess endlessly about its symbolism. I'll begin to worry about my health to the point where I can't look at my hand without noticing the arch of the blue stripe of vein under the skin, and the pulse beating steadily within it. Against my own will I'll imagine the blood passing through those tunnels and I'll sense each individual cell careening through, wondering if they are all right, or if, against all odds, something evil is brewing inside there again.

And then there are the funeral parlors, with their gracious awnings and the glow of soft lamplight from within. For years after my illness I would cross the street to avoid walking past one. I felt them calling to me. I felt that their energy was drawing me in, like a slow-moving but irresistible whirlpool, against whose steady pressure there was no defense. I began to imagine that my image might be posted inside, on a "most wanted" list, issued by the Association of the Angels of

Death, and that if I crossed too close I might be recognized and picked up for bounty.

As I go on and on while others drop off the face of the Earth with regularity, as the casualties mount around me, the impact of each unfathomable confrontation with death grows increasingly strong and constant. It is knowledge I would erase from my psyche in an instant if I could. Yet every so often, it is that knowledge that lifts me above any exaltation I have ever known.

When I'm suffering through my periods of difficulty, when I find myself locked away from the appreciation I know I should feel in my journey through this life, I'm always aware of a little doorway that exists down near the floor of my conciousness. It's a doorway that I never open without great effort, and most times I only succeed at crouching low and peeking through. But when I do open the door and bend down to its level, I feel like Alice after she passed through the looking glass. A giant peering into a world I'm much too clumsy to inhabit. It's the world where all my concerns carry no weight, and where nothing that has caught hold of me in recent years has any sway over my soul. It's the land that I inhabited when all I craved was a day free from pain, and when I knew how to cherish such a luxury. Even more occasionally I can, through means I don't fully understand, pass easily through the doorway, and play like a child on the other side. Those are the moments of my life. The moments I thought my life would forever after be. The quickest way — sometimes the only way — to conjure one of those moments, is to have a brush with death.

I've heard it said that whatever doesn't kill you makes you stronger. I've also heard it said that whatever doesn't kill you fucks you up for a really long time, and it's a miracle if you ever get it back together again. I have a great doctor now. Her name is Julia. Julia is a very attractive, warm, energetic woman who is not so very much older than I am. I see her every few months, just for a checkup, and every time I do, she loves to tease me about a TV sitcom that I once made.

"Oh, boy! Did that stink," she says, every time I see her.

On a recent visit I told her, "Hey. That TV show has allowed me to turn down quite a few other things already." And I started to tell her about a play that I had just turned down that day. Not because it wasn't any good, I just couldn't get excited about it. "It's a lot of work," I said. "If it doesn't mean something to me, personally, I don't want to spend my time on it."

I told her that I had been writing about the illness, and about a passage where I talk about "spending time." How I want to "spend" my days. I said, "I've become a miser, Julia. I don't want to give them away. I want to possess my time. Hoard it, save it up, and collect interest on it. The more time that I keep for myself, the more the interest will build up, and my time collection will grow and grow and grow."

I expected her to laugh at me for being such a sensitive, artistic type who's afraid of hard work. Instead she looked into my eyes, and she said, "That's great. You've been through a lot. Your perspective has changed. That's a good thing. You don't know how long you're going to be around — no one knows how many years they've got — but you've learned that better than most people ever have to. You should only do what you want to be doing with those moments."

I said, "No, Julia. No. Nothing's changed. I mean, I sure don't wake up every morning just thrilled to be alive, not needing anything else, like I swore I would when I was sick. No. Most of the time, I'm just . . . sad, about everything that happened, and how much it cost me."

I told her how, after I got well from the transplant, for a long time, I couldn't get myself to get up off the couch. I had my health back, but I didn't feel like *doing anything*. I just felt, well — if my life doesn't depend on it, why bother?

"But that doesn't last," I said. "Because when that play opens, I'm going to be jealous of whoever's in it. Even though I wasn't willing to give up my time to do it. See, I still want to be in that race, on some level. To compete, just for the sake of the competition. So maybe what I mean is, well . . . yes. Everything's changed. But then, it all becomes the same again."

Julia said, "Of course. There's an innocence in that. In that race. In being able to believe in that. And that's a very painful loss you've suffered, the loss of that innocence."

And we walked out of the examination room, down a narrow hallway stacked with medical records. Julia had her hand resting on my back, between the shoulder blades. She gave me two pats on the back, and as she pushed me toward the door she said, "You take care — *Old Man.*"

I left the doctor's office laughing, and took the elevator down to the first floor. I left the building, and I walked out, into a delicious, refreshing, cold winter rain.

ENDNOTE

While this book accurately reflects the state of advanced medical treatments during the mid- to late nineteen-eighties, many develop-ments since then have already altered the landscape. Primarily, in the arena of bone marrow transplantation, the advent of "growth-stimulating factors" — drugs that can selectively stimulate the regen-eration of specific marrow-cell lines — has substantially lowered the mortality risk from infection. Since the stimulating factors can reduce the patient's neutrapoenic period, many bacterial and/or viral infec-tions can be either avoided or limited in their duration and severity. At the time of this writing, the mortality rate from infection during bone marrow transplantation at top facilities was inching below 3 percent — not much higher than the risk associated with coronary bypass surgery. As the understanding of genetic and cellular science continues to improve, it is reasonable to hope that the treatments involved in bone marrow transplantation will continue to improve as well. Eventually, perhaps, such drastic treatments will be ren-dered unnecessary.